RIVKA LEVY

TALK TO GOD
AND FIX YOUR HEALTH

The three main reasons why we're really getting sick.

How to identify and defuse messy emotional issues
before they turn into physical illnesses.

Easy ways to fix your health at the spiritual,
emotional and physical levels.

**Best of all, the ideas in the book actually work,
and can lead to dramatic, fast and permanent
improvements to your health.**

The Real Reasons Why We Get Sick and How to Stay Healthy

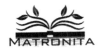

MATRONITA

Levy, Rivka
Talk to God and Fix Your Health / Rivka Levy – First edition
ISBN: Trade Paperback: 978-965-7739-01-3
ISBN: eBook: 978-965-7739-04-4
FIRST EDITION
Printed in the USA

For R, M, and T

May God continue to keep us healthy and
happy all the long days of our lives

Midreshet B'erot Bat Ayin
The Village of Bat Ayin
Gush Etzion, Israel 90913

מדרשת בארות בת עין
ישוב בת עין 90913
ישראל

Talk to G-d And Fix Your Health by Rivka Levy takes you on a healing journey to unblock negative emotions and unhealthy habits in order to "defuse your emotional issues before they turn into physical illnesses." As the title of the book testifies, Rivka Levy demonstrates how all health and healing ultimately emanates from G-d. The essence of achieving and maintaining good health is to ingest G- dJuice through talking to G-d regularly, cultivating positive thinking and gratefulness as well as developing healthy compassion, sensible accounting and appropriate kindness. The author explains each concept in a very easily read book full of life examples and peppered with energy healing exercises. When reading this innovative book you will feel like Rivka is talking directly to you about her own healing process. She incorporates her vast knowledge of the meridians with their emotional and physical issues, as well as an extensive explanation of how to identify negative influences and overcome them. The book is especially helpful for those who are looking for ways out of loneliness, disconnection, despair and depression. May *Talk to G-d and Fix Your Health* reach many readers who will benefit from its uplifting healing message!

    With Blessings of the Torah & the Land,

    Chana Bracha Siegelbaum

    Chana Bracha Siegelbaum

Founder and Director of *Midreshet B'erot Bat Ayin: Holistic Torah for Women on the Land* and author of several books including the award-winning book *The Seven Fruits of the Land of Israel with their Mystical and Medicinal Properties.*

'When prayer is liberated and redeemed, all doctors and medical treatment will become redundant'

Rebbe Nachman of Breslev, Likutey Moharan 2, 1:9

CONTENTS

ACKNOWLEDGEMENTS

There came a point, after I'd been working on this manuscript for more than a year, that it seemed as though it was never going to see the light of day. My computer died, taking with it all my 'Talk to God and Fix Your Health' writings and source material.

Even though I was convinced that this book had the potential to transform the issue of health and well-being for large numbers of people, when that happened I bowed to the seemingly inevitable, grieved for the book, and got ready to throw the computer out.

My husband rescued my laptop from the rubbish bin (or 'garbage pail,' for American readers) and decided to try one more time to get it to work, including changing the plug.

Miracle of miracles! The computer – and my book manuscript – sprang back to life. But I'd lost my enthusiasm for the whole project, so the book still sat dormant for another two months, until my friend and chief cheerleader, Sarah Prais, encouraged me to get it finished.

Without her helpful nagging, you wouldn't be reading this.

Two other Sarahs helped bring this book to fruition: Sarah (Sacha) Levein, who undertook the mammoth task of reading the first version, and Sarah McNamara, who edited the manuscript to perfection. I also want to thank Raphael Albinati for bringing his superb design talents to bear on this book.

The greatest acknowledgement of all has to be to God, who pulled off a number of miraculous feats in order to get this book out of my head, and into your hands, not least, continuing to shine His light when all around me was darkness.

I hope that I captured at least some of that light in these pages, and that this book will help to illuminate other people's path towards true happiness, self-fulfillment, and radiant good health.

Rivka Levy

Jerusalem, 2015

Introduction

The Missing Link

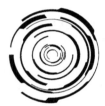

Staying happy and healthy is probably one of the most important goals for pretty much every single person on the planet. Everyone knows that nothing can impact your joy and quality of life like serious, chronic, emotional and physical illnesses.

Unfortunately, staying fit and healthy isn't always so easy or straightforward. For example, many people believe that diet and exercise are the key to good health - and it's certainly true that high-quality food and appropriate exercise can work wonders, for your body and mood. But it's not quite the whole story.

What about all of those people who religiously ate their steamed veggies and brown rice for years, or who were world-class athletes on super-strict, super-healthy diets - who still went on to develop a whole bunch of nasty diseases?

Or at the other end of the scale, what about all those people who religiously eat their Big Mac and fries every single day, wash it down with a Coke or beer, and finish up by chain-smoking a few cigarettes - and they live in good health to over 100!?

Clearly, good food and exercise is an important component of staying healthy, but it's not the whole picture.

So what's missing?

Let's switch sides, from body to soul, to see if there's an answer on that side of the equation. Many complementary and alternative health practitioners are well-versed on the more spiritual and energetic dimension to health.

They'll tell you all about how important your body's energetic vibrations are; give you a million-and-one techniques for keeping your aura strong, and advise you to get in tune with your 'inner child' and your spirit, and to do the deep inner work you need to heal, emotionally and physically.

Again, this is all really good stuff, generally speaking, but it's still not the whole picture of how to stay healthy.

You can be sniffing your tailored aromatherapy blend, sleeping with your crystals and doing yoga until the cows come home - and still get sick. You can also still suffer from anxiety, stress and depression, as well as all sorts of other physical illnesses and problems. Clearly, energy work in all its forms is an important part of staying healthy, but it's not the whole jalapeno.

But what about conventional medicine? Maybe obediently taking the drugs you're being prescribed by your doctor, and undergoing all the surgical procedures they recommend, from minor to major, is the best way to maintain your health? A quick look at the latest medical statistics shows that there are many problems inherent in this approach to health too, as between 100,000 - 300,000 people a year are dying from taking their medications *as prescribed.*

Even when you regularly go to your doctors, and you regularly take your pills, and you obediently have your surgeries, you can still stay sick.

So what's the answer? What's missing from the whole health equation? Is it really possible to live stress-free, emotionally happy and physically healthy lives?

The answer is: yes, but only if you've got enough GodJuice flowing through your system, and you really understand which factors are truly affecting your health and well-being.

If you're drinking your green smoothies and cleansing your auras, or swallowing your pills and going for your annual check-ups - but God is absent from your picture - then you're missing a massive part of your health care puzzle.

When you have enough GodJuice in your life, you usually find it much easier to make and maintain the changes you need to stay physically and emotionally healthy. You tend to eat healthier, act nicer, and live a longer, more productive life.

You also start to internalize that your illnesses and health challenges aren't just random occurrences, or caused by genes or germs, they are actually part of the conversation God is trying to have with every single one of us.

Over the coming pages, you're going to learn how the 'Talk to God and Fix Your Health' approach holds the key to creating a successful blueprint for emotional and physical health. It's much easier than you think, and I *guarantee* that if you try to implement the approach set out in this book, you'll see huge, positive changes in every area of your life.

Of course, you can still eat your sprouts and take your vitamins in the meantime. The 'Talk to God' approach works with every other health system out there, and it's not an all or nothing deal. The key thing to remember is that no matter what you're doing to stay healthy, if you're starting out with enough GodJuice, it'll be that much more effective, long-lasting and profound.

GodJuice is the crucial ingredient that will make the single biggest positive impact on your health and well-being, as you're about to find out over the coming pages.

Chapter 1

Why You Need GodJuice In Order To Feel Good

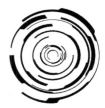

Let's start with a working definition of what GodJuice actually is:

> *GodJuice is that feeling you get when your soul is healthy and happy, you feel powered-up and connected to God, and you're full of energy, motivation and life.*

When your soul gets disconnected from God, it's like a laptop that's gone for too long away from its power source. Sure, it's got some battery reserves that can keep it going for a while, but sooner or later if it doesn't get a top up of GodJuice, it's going to go to sleep (or even shut down completely, God forbid).

Just like the laptop starts to slow up and freeze as it starts to power-down, that's what happens to a human being when it doesn't have enough GodJuice.

When you don't have enough GodJuice, the world becomes an incredibly scary, dark and frightening place. I mean, have you listened to the news lately? Do you know how many wars are going on, how bad the economy really is, how many dangerous psychopaths are on the prowl in your neighborhood?

It's enough to give anyone a heart attack...

When you don't have enough GodJuice, the world becomes this random, meaningless place where anything can happen to anyone, for any reason or no reason at all.

- You could randomly get Ebola from the person you sit next to on the bus...

- You could get all bitter and beat yourself up for the next 50 years that the ONE time you didn't buy a ticket, your numbers came up on the lottery...

- You could get really down and depressed any time even the smallest little thing doesn't go your way...

- You could fly into an ulcer-inducing fit of rage when your defiant teenager fails to give you respect and do as you say...

- You could worry yourself to death about how you're going to pay all the bills due at the end of the month, with your teeny-tiny salary...

- You could get into a serious car crash any time you hit the road...

If you really stop to think about it, the number of bad things that could potentially happen to you every single day is mind-boggling. The world is full of uncertainty; you have no guarantees that you're going to make it through the next five minutes in one piece, let alone the next 100 years.

It's such a scary thought that most people are trying to do anything they can to avoid thinking about it: they party hard, they work hard, they fill their lives up with hobbies, social events, sports and entertainment. Why are they doing all this? Because they don't have enough GodJuice.

Once you start to boost your GodJuice, all the madness in the world, and all the apparent meanness and suffering stops being so scary. Of course, that doesn't automatically mean that you're always going to understand what's going on, but the thought that there is 'Someone' in charge, even when your life starts to fall apart at the seams, is profoundly comforting, on a soul level.

> *The more investment you put into pumping up*
> *your GodJuice, the safer you'll start to feel.*

Let's take all the worry and fear you currently feel about catching Ebola. Your anxiety about Ebola is closing down your spiritual, emotional and physical circuits. As soon as you give it to God to deal with, your energetic, emotional and spiritual blocks will disappear, and you'll be able to re-access all the GodJuice you need to function. You'll start feeling happier, significantly less worried and anxious, and you'll start sleeping better, too. Your tension headaches will disappear, and you'll start enjoying your outings to the mall again.

But if you don't try to give all of your fears and worries about 'what might be' with the Ebola virus back to God, then what can happen?

- Your GodJuice can plummet, and you start to feel weak, overwhelmed and incredibly anxious;

- You start to get paranoid;

- When someone sneezes anywhere near you, your heartbeat doubles and your blood pressure shoots through the roof;

- You get angry if someone coughs in your direction, or even comes close enough to breathe on you;

- You buy a face mask and actually start wearing it around;

- You start turning down social invitations and turn into a hermit;

- You can lose all your friends;

- You can lose your job;

- You can get all down and depressed about the miserable state your life is in, on top of still being paranoid about catching Ebola.

And so on, and so forth.

You can sum it up this way:

When you have low or depleted GodJuice, it's just a matter of time before you start to develop a whole bunch of negative emotions, stress and worries, which can, in turn, lead to a whole slew of physical problems and challenges. That's why the more GodJuice you have, the healthier you'll be.

GOD IS BEHIND EVERYTHING

While this idea can sound incredibly radical to people used to Western medicine, and its strict separation between the body and the soul, spiritually speaking it makes perfect sense.

While it's relatively easy to ignore social problems, children problems, marital problems, money problems - all big clues that God might be sending you to encourage you to change something in your life, behavior, beliefs or outlook - as soon as you get sick, you tend to notice really fast, and react immediately.

Western medicine only starts to deal with 'the problem,' whatever it is, once it's already manifested as a specific physical or mental health issue or illness. Energy Medicine, including acupuncture, acupressure and other forms of traditional Chinese Medicine, starts to deal with the problem at the 'energetic' level, when it starts to disrupt the energy flowing through the body.

But the 'Talk to God' approach set out in this book goes back a stage further, and starts to treat the problem at its source. If you can keep your GodJuice healthy and humming, you can usually manage to avoid most of the problems heading your way before they even turn into something concrete.

How can you do that? Read on!

The 'Talk to God and Fix Your Health' program can be broken down into a few main founding principles, as follows:

The First Principle: Recharge Your GodJuice Every Day

The single best way to keep your GodJuice healthy is to talk to God every single day. I'll tell you more about this a little later, but don't let the simplicity of this idea blind you to its power: it can literally transform your life and your health, overnight, when you know how to apply it properly.

The Second Principle: Work On Your Negative Emotions

This may come as a surprise to some people, but your negative emotions don't just disappear by themselves the older you get; in fact, the opposite is usually true. The next thing that's usually making you sick, sad and depressed, (once you've taken care of your weak or chronically-depleted GodJuice) are your negative emotions. Any effort you make to work on your negative emotions, and to clean them out of your system, will pay out massive, lasting dividends for maintaining your mental and physical health.

Throughout this book, I'll share some effective, easy tools and exercises with you that can help you to clean up your emotional act, fast.

When you act like a jerk - when you steal, lie, cheat or hurt someone else with your cruel or selfish behavior - your GodJuice gets completely whacked out, and your negative emotions go berserk.

That's the bad news.

The first of many pieces of good news that you'll find in this book is that it's actually really easy to fix all this stuff, get your GodJuice back up to speed and your negative emotions back under control. Here's how:

1. Own up to doing whatever bad thing you did, and admit that it was wrong;

2. Apologize in whatever way you need to;

3. Ask God to help you fix it, so you don't do it again.

That's it! Now your GodJuice is flowing again, and you'll have the inner strength and fortitude you need to get back on top of your negative emotions, and to stop them from ruining your life, mood and health.

The second piece of good news is that you don't have to fix everything at once. If you make an effort to catch even one thing, every single day, that's enough to boost your GodJuice, and to get all the other bad stuff cleaned out of your system, over time. God wants you to try, to start the process off, but He'll do the rest.

We'll come back to the idea of what 'acting nice' actually means a little later on, but for now, it's enough to know that you shouldn't act nice because it's the right thing to do, you should act nice because it's going to make *you* happy and healthy.

Generous, kind, thoughtful people tend to have much more GodJuice coursing through their body, and tend to be much healthier than people who are full of fear, anger, worry, jealousy and other negative emotions.

The Third Principle: Take Stock of Where You're Really Holding

We'll cover this in more detail when you get to the chapter on how to develop Sensible Accountability, but when you do things wrong, and you don't make an effort to clean them up and say sorry for them (both to God and to the people you may have hurt or upset) - this seriously depletes your GodJuice and can kill your spiritual energy.

Dodgy business deals, rage fits you had at your kids, flipping the bird at the guy who stole your parking spot - all these things severely affect your GodJuice, and can also have a huge impact on your energy and your health.

Trouble is, most of us do a lot of these sorts of things on autopilot without even thinking about it. Or if you do happen to think about it, it's easy enough to find justifications and excuses for why it was really *okay*. That's why it's crucially important to spend at least a minute or two a day trying to go through this stuff as dispassionately and objectively as you can.

Again, you aren't taking stock of where you're really holding because it's the right thing to do (even though it is); you're trying to take stock of where you're really holding because you want to catch the events, reactions and emotions that might be taking out your GodJuice, and making you much more vulnerable to developing an emotional or physical illness.

As you'll learn a little later on, trying to shove all these things under the carpet because you don't really have the time, energy or inclination to deal with them only backfires in the long run. If you don't address this stuff while it's still at the level of being a spiritual, energetic or emotional problem, sooner or later it will show up as a physical health issue that you just can't ignore anymore.

Your body and soul are intricately and inseparably connected; if there's a problem in one, it will be reflected in the other, and vice versa. The more 'junk' emotions and attitudes there are hiding away in your soul, for example, the more you'll be attracted to 'junk' in the physical, material world; like junk food, alcohol, cigarettes, and internet porn.

GodJuice helps you to stay fit and well, because it keeps your soul healthy, which in turn is reflected in a fit, strong, healthy body.

The Fourth Principle: GodJuice Is Not All or Nothing

Keeping your GodJuice flowing is a lifelong process, and it's definitely not all or nothing. One day, you can be on top of the world, and see the GodJuice in every tiny thing in your life. The very next day, (and occasionally, even the very next hour or minute) you can literally fall down a deep, dark hole, and have no idea what on earth's going on, or where God is meant to be hiding Himself in the big mess called 'your life.'

God knows that you're not always going to pass the tests He's sending you. He knows that occasionally, as hard as you try, you just can't see past the person that's annoying you, or pretend that you're really happy about what's occurring in your life when really, you're not. He understands that sometimes you don't have the first clue about what you're meant to be trying to change or fix in your life, and that you also don't have the energy to start trying to work it all out.

That's because you're a human being, not a robot.

The good news is God loves you unconditionally. As long as you're continuing to strive to get closer to God, even when you can't see Him, or can't find Him, you can be sure that your efforts will ultimately be rewarded in the most amazing way, and that you will blossom into the happy, healthy, emotionally beautiful person that God created you to be.

Putting it into practice

In this book, you're going to learn many practical tools and powerful techniques for boosting your GodJuice; detoxing your body and soul, overcoming negative emotions and solving the riddle of why you may be getting sick. But before you read on, I have to tell you the secret of how you can turn all this theoretical advice into concrete improvements in your own life:

> *Work on boosting your GodJuice every single day.*

If you get God involved in implementing the ideas in this book, and you start to talk to Him for at least five minutes a day, you'll see all sorts of things moving and shifting in your life. And what if you don't? Depending on your willpower and determination, you may well see some things move a bit. But the changes you'll experience without God are unlikely to completely transform your life in the same way; they're unlikely to last very long and they're unlikely to lead to true happiness, inner peace and optimal good health.

So the first powerful tool for achieving real health and well-being is this:

> *Get God involved in your life in practice and not just in theory.*

The Fifth Principle: GodJuice Is for Everyone

You don't have to be 'religious' to work on developing your GodJuice. GodJuice is non-denominational, and it works for anyone, anywhere, at any time.

Many people, 'religious' or otherwise, like to think that they already have all the GodJuice they need in their lives, and they might even be right! But there's one way to tell for sure: when you genuinely do have a healthy amount of GodJuice flowing through your veins, you're usually very happy. Specifically that means that you're happy with your lot in life, including every little small detail of it, right down to your problems and 'lacks.'

Again, let's try to step away from the theory, and put it into practical terms.

If you want to know if you're really filled up with GodJuice, go through the following checklist, and see how many of them apply to you:

- You're generally happy with yourself - including your appearance, personality, 'essence,' health issues, family circumstances, finances, successes and failures.

- You're generally happy with your spouse (and not beating yourself up for not marrying the other guy who proposed in college...)

- You're generally happy with your kids - even the ones you sometimes don't like very much because they're getting into trouble at school / wetting the bed every night / or are otherwise 'difficult' to deal with.

- You're happy with your home, financial status, and bank account - even if you're drowning in debt, or don't have a home, or don't have any financial assets.

- You're happy with your family circumstances - even if you grew up with the worst parents ever, and you're still trying to deal with the fallout.

- You have no complaints about your life, or the way God is running your particular show.

Genuinely being this happy takes a lot of work, a lot of GodJuice, and an awful lot of Heavenly help. That's why it's IMPOSSIBLE to really be happy and healthy, unless your GodJuice is humming. That's also why your happiness is such a good barometer of how much GodJuice you really do have.

A Reminder: How GodJuice is directly connected to your health and well-being

When you don't have enough GodJuice, you get miserable, stressed and ill. A stressed, miserable person doesn't eat right and doesn't sleep right, and is full of negative emotions, anxiety and other bad characteristics like anger, jealousy and self-pity.

In turn, these negative emotions can - and do - back up in your physical and energetic systems, where they can cause all sorts of physical and emotional health issues, if they aren't properly dealt with and addressed.

Miracle cures

I know that these ideas can sound a little strange to those of us who grew up with the Western medical model that germs (or accidents) are responsible for all sickness and death.

For now, let me just tell you that there are countless stories of medical miracles that happened when people stopped relying on doctors, or whatever other man-made crutch they were using, and started working on their GodJuice instead. Terminal diseases disappeared overnight, holes in the heart closed up and chronic diseases vanished.

We'll come back to this topic in much more detail a little later on, in Chapter 10. Let's end by recapping what you just learned in this chapter.

RECAP

- When you don't have enough GodJuice, you can get stressed, worried, anxious and develop a whole range of negative emotions that, in turn, can make you physically ill.

- GodJuice is not all-or-nothing: it's a constant process of growth and self-discovery that continues throughout your life.

- If you're genuinely happy being you, warts n' all, you'll have a very high level of GodJuice flowing through your body. If your GodJuice is low, then you'll have a predisposition to feel unsatisfied, frustrated and unhappy with your life and circumstances, even if they're objectively wonderful.

- The more you power-up your GodJuice, the happier and healthier you'll be.

Chapter 2

How to Get Your GodJuice Humming

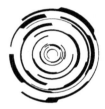

The single best way to maximize your GodJuice is to talk to God on a regular basis, preferably every single day.

Now, I know that's a big deal, and a big commitment, but here's the deal: if you don't put God in the picture, nothing else you do, health-wise, is going to work so well. Yes, I know it often *appears* as though all the other tools for dealing with anxiety, depression, anger, or physical illnesses work just fine by themselves, but if you look closer, you'll see that it's actually not true.

Let's take a few common examples: Mr A takes the medication prescribed by his doctor to deal with his depression and anxiety – and ends up with a slew of other problems to deal with, including loss of libido, weight gain and problems sleeping. Why? Because the medication upset the careful balance in Mr A's bio-chemistry, leading to a bunch of other health issues and problems.

The problem didn't really get resolved, it just got shifted downstream.

Or, let's say Mrs B goes the therapy route to try to deal with her chronic anger. She believes her horrible boss is the trigger for her rage attacks, and spends months and maybe even years working it through with her therapist. At the end of the process, she can handle her boss amazingly well – but now her kids are driving her up the wall.

Why? Because without God in the picture, you often get stuck on the externals, or symptoms of the problem, without really getting close to their inner dimension.

This applies to any healing art you care to mention, from surgery to acupuncture to tapping to Energy Medicine – and everything else in between. Either the solution doesn't work at all, or it doesn't work so well, or the 'problem' just pops up in some other place, instead.

Why is this?

This happens because the real root of all of your emotional and physical problems is spiritual, i.e., God is causing you difficulties in order to get you to change or fix something in yourself and in your life. When you really start living the reality that God is behind every single detail in your life, from the smallest to the largest, from the cuddliest and cutest to the scariest - that's when you'll truly start to find fast, permanent and effective cures to all of your emotional and physical health issues.

Defusing negative emotions

As you spend more time talking to God about what's really going on in your life and inside your head, negative emotions like fear, anxiety, anger and hatred can start to disappear pretty fast. But that doesn't meant that you're always going to be instantly happy about everything that happens to you, or that these negative emotions will simply vanish in a puff of smoke, never to return.

Like most things of value, permanently defusing your negative emotions is a process that can last a pretty long time. Even if you've been working on your GodJuice for a while, you'll probably still freak out when you hear about the latest terrorist attack; you'll probably still feel panic when your husband gets laid off at work; and you'll probably still hate the old friend who stabbed you in the back - but instead of stewing over that stuff for weeks, months or even years, now you'll be able to take all those disturbing things back to God.

When you do that on a regular basis, you'll find that God starts helping you to clear out all those negative experiences, reactions and feelings much faster, so they don't get a chance to bed in and do some permanent damage to your health and well-being.

Once you start talking to God on a regular basis, instead of panicking for three days, you'll just panic for three minutes. Instead of feeling like you're going to throw up from nerves, you'll just feel a bit dry-mouthed. Instead of being unable to sleep for months, you'll have one rough night, discuss it with God the next day, and then feel so much better.

Regular doses of GodJuice help you to detox your soul from negative feelings and bad characteristics for the following reasons:

1) God Can Actually Solve Your Problems

A great reason for talking to God is that He can actually help you solve all your problems in life.

If you're struggling to put food on the table, or you're trying to move country or city, or you're dealing with a seriously ill relative, that issue is still going to cause you a lot of physical stress and difficulty, no matter what you're trying to do to calm yourself down and to cope with it all.

But when you talk to God about it all, it doesn't just make you feel better because you have a shoulder to cry on, it can also *solve your problem for you*, when nothing else can. Stories abound of people getting miracle cures, miracle money and miracle solutions after they spent even just a little bit of time working on their GodJuice.

2) It Helps You Work Out What's Really Going On In Your Head

As we mentioned earlier, most people have a blind spot when it comes to identifying their own flaws, bad behavior and inappropriate reactions. When you make an effort to talk to God about the stuff that's going on in your life, it helps you to develop more objectivity about what you may need to work on, or change about yourself.

3) You Get a Lot of Heavenly Help to Find Solutions to Your Problems

When you get God involved in finding a solution to your problems, health-related or otherwise, you can be sure that the solutions you discover will be fast, easy and effective. When you don't get God involved, you can end up going around in circles for years, fruitlessly trying to resolve your anger problem or your anxiety problem without ever really discovering the true cause of your negative emotions.

As the old adage goes, an accurate diagnosis is more than half the cure.

So without any further ado, let's learn how you can tap into your very own reservoir of GodJuice and get it working for you.

How to pray for your mental and physical health in a way that's scientifically proven to work:

Over the decades, a number of scientific experiments have been carried out by medical researchers to test the therapeutic effects of prayer. *(The following quotations are from 'Healing Words' by Larry Dossey, MD, which cites a number of these experiments.)*

In the first experiment, researchers at the Spindrift research lab in Oregon used an alcohol rinse to half-kill a mold culture they were growing. Then, they put a string down the middle of the culture dish, and asked half their volunteers to pray in a 'directed' way for side A of the mold, (i.e., requesting a specific outcome) and the other volunteers were asked to pray in a 'non-directed' way for side B (i.e., simply requesting whatever outcome would be best, without specifying it).

Nothing much happened on side A, but the mold on side B started multiplying at a rate of knots, and quickly sprang back to life.

In repeated experiments, the Spindrift researchers found that: "prayer works, and that both methods are effective. But...the non-directed technique appeared quantitatively more effective, *frequently yielding results that were twice as great, or more, when compared to the directed approach*" (emphasis mine).

Hold on to that piece of information; I'll explain its relevance to your life and your issues in a minute. But before I do, let me tell you about a second experiment, this time conducted at the University of Redlands in 1951.

A group of 45 volunteers with a range of physical and mental issues were divided into three groups, of 15 people each. The first was called: 'Just-Plain-Psychology,' the second: 'Just-Plain-Prayer' and the last group was called: 'Prayer Therapy Group'.

In the first group, no one mentioned religion or prayer, it was just straight-up psychotherapy, as the patients in this group had indicated they wanted.

In the second group, no one mentioned therapy. It consisted of a bunch of practicing 'true believers,' who already thought they knew how to pray, and that prayer was all they needed to get well. This group spent every night for nine months praying that *God would cure them of their specific illness or emotional problem* (emphasis mine).

The last group combined two-hour weekly prayer sessions with psychological testing. Each week, participants in this group got an envelope telling them about a negative aspect of their personality that the therapists had identified, and asked them to pray for help on eliminating it.

After nine months, the results of the experiment were as follows:

1. **Just Therapy Group: 65% improvement.**

2. **Just Prayer Group:** *No improvement.*

3. **Prayer and Psychological Testing: 72% improvement.**

These results puzzled and even disturbed many 'religious' people at the time - but by the time you've finished reading this book, they'll make perfect sense.

The first thing to remember is what you just learned above, namely that you can't force God to give you exactly what you want. That's why non-directed prayer - where you pray for your general good, as opposed to a specific outcome - is far more effective than asking for something concrete.

The second thing to remember is that *God only sends you your illnesses as a wake-up call, to get you to change or fix something in yourself, life, relationships or beliefs.*

Groups I and III were actively working on themselves, albeit in different ways, and were making changes in response to their illness or issue. To put it another way, a large majority of them successfully got the message that God was sending them via their illness, so the illness itself become surplus to Divine requirements.

By contrast, those in Group II weren't working on anything, nor were they apparently willing to change anything, so their illnesses and issues remained the same at the end of the nine months as they had been at the beginning.

In addition, this group was praying specifically for God to take away their illness or issue (which is 'directed' prayer), as opposed to asking God to do whatever was best for them ('non-directed' prayer).

So what can you learn from all of these scientific experiments about what really works when it comes to praying for your health and well-ness? Let's try to sum it up:

1. Don't ask God to 'take away' your specific health problem ('directed' prayer); instead, ask God to do whatever's best for you ('non-directed' prayer).

2. Be prepared to change something in yourself or your life if you want to get well - because the illness is only coming to give you a message. Once you get the message - and act on it - nine times out of 10, the physical and / or emotional illness will vanish by itself.

3. Prayer really works - and its success rate is often much greater than more conventional therapeutic techniques and approaches.

How to get your GodJuice flowing

This can be as simple, or as complicated as you care to make it. You can talk to God for just a minute a day, or literally spend the whole day thrashing things out with Him (and believe it or not, there are people who do this on a regular basis).

When you start off trying to talk to God, you shouldn't worry too much about what you're saying, or how you're trying to say it. Just as a baby's first words are so precious and treasured and celebrated by their parents - even though fundamentally, all they said was 'Mommy' - that's exactly how it is when you start talking to God.

God knows that you feel like the world's biggest idiot, the first time you make the effort to try to talk to Him, but He's still giving you His full attention. All you have to do is turn the tap on for the GodJuice to start flowing, and then just wait for the right words to show up, and for your conversations to get longer, easier, more meaningful and insightful, and more helpful, as you go along.

In the meantime, even if you only manage to say one sincere word every other month, that one word is still moving mountains for you, spiritually. Even if you only manage to talk to God truthfully just once in your life, it will count for more than you can ever begin to fathom.

So, especially when you're starting out, it doesn't really matter how much you talk to God, or what you say, or how long you spend doing it. But that said, there are still some broad guidelines for how you can make the most of your time talking to God.

THE EIGHT SECRETS OF BOOSTING YOUR GODJUICE

1)   Start Small

It's much better to get a regular shot of GodJuice for just five minutes, every single day, than to try to kick off with a whole day-long GodJuice extravaganza. Consistency and persistency nearly always lead to better results than show-stopping one-offs.

2)   Don't Censor Yourself

Tell God everything that's on your mind. For GodJuice to work, it has to be honest. If you've learned that you're not meant to complain about anything, but you're still feeling really angry, tell God that! He knows anyway, so your fake piety isn't winning you any prizes. GodJuice is much more about owning up to your ugly truths than trying to present your beautiful lies.

3)   Don't Pressure Yourself to Say Anything

Especially at the beginning. God gives the words, and God gives the silence. Sometimes, the silence is exactly what you need, as it could be the first time you're actually giving your inner dimension some time to express itself. It's amazing what you can learn about yourself when you finally turn off all the 'noise' that's blaring in your head.

4)   GodJuice Isn't Just About Talking - It's Also About Listening

Yes, tell God about everything that's on your mind, thank Him for all the great stuff He's doing for you, ask Him for help - and then pay attention to what God is telling *you*. This is where some amazing changes can happen, but only if you're really listening out for the insights that God's going to give you.

That doesn't mean that you'll literally hear God conducting a conversation with you, (if that happens to you, it's either really, really good, or really, really bad...) but God talks to you all the time via your environment, experiences and thoughts. The trick is to tune out your intellect, and tune into your soul, to really hear what He's trying to tell you.

5)   Do It by Yourself

If you've never tried GodJuice before, then trying to do it when you're sitting on the bench at your local park along with 500 other people around may not be the best way to start. Go for a solitary walk somewhere pretty, sit in your garden, or do it for a few minutes in bed when you wake up. You'll get over the 'feeling stupid' effect much faster if you're by yourself and not worrying that someone else is watching while you're apparently 'talking to yourself.'

6)   Don't Give Up!

GodJuice is a learning process. I've had days when it was fabulous, days when it came very hard, and days when I spent most of the time just repeating 'God is all there is' because I was too shell-shocked to say anything else. God loves your effort, and He's happy to hear whatever comes out of your mouth (or doesn't even...). The more you work on your GodJuice, the more safe, happy, optimistic and confident you'll start to feel, even if you're having trouble just stringing basic sentences together.

You just need to show up. God will do the rest.

7)   Get God Involved In Your Healing Process

If you don't get God involved in your healing process, then most of what you'll learn in this book will remain at the level of being an intellectual exercise. But if you start talking to God about the changes you want to see happen, both in your emotional and physical health, and in your life generally, then the sky is really the limit. When God is involved, a huge amount of personal growth and change is possible, even in a relatively short amount of time.

8)   Say Thank You

If you really want to see fast results, the strongest brand of GodJuice I know is to say thank you for your problems. I know this sounds counter-intuitive - maybe even dumb - but let me explain why this could be one of the most effective strategies for turning your biggest problems around, fast.

It's human nature to moan and complain, and to feel sorry for yourself, but nothing dries up your GodJuice as fast, or as fundamentally, as complaining and whining. When you tell God 'thanks' for all the stuff going on in your life, even the bad stuff, even the huge, apparently unsolvable health problem you're dealing with, it's a massive spiritual shortcut, and it blows all the spiritual blockages to smithereens.

Saying 'thank you' can get the GodJuice pumping again, like nothing else.

It's not easy to do - but it works. I've heard more stories than I can count about people who said thank you for their tumors - and the cancer disappeared. Or people who said thank you for their chronic illnesses and autoimmune diseases, and they literally disappeared overnight.

Energetically, gratitude is one of the most powerful healing forces in the body. When it's combined with GodJuice, it can become an unstoppable, even miraculous, force for health and well-being.

To give just one example, in his book 'Gratitude Works,' Robert Emmons explains how adopting an attitude of gratitude has been scientifically proven to boost your health in a number of ways, including enabling you to cope with, and bounce back from stress much easier.

How to implement the stuff in this book

Let me ask you something: How many self-help books have you already read? How many New Year's resolutions have you already made to change, or improve, or to do things differently? After all the classes you've taken, and all the stuff you've already learned, and all the efforts you've already made, how much did your life actually change?

As I mentioned earlier, GodJuice is the key to taking the things you're learning in this book (and anything else you want to learn and implement) out of the realm of 'theory,' and putting it into practice.

When you don't talk to God about your issues, difficulties, and health problems, very little of substance normally changes. You can read all the self-help books you want, learn all the inspiring spiritual ideas out there, buy all the chia seeds, and drink all the green smoothies known to man - but you still often won't have the courage and ability required to follow through with your truth, and make the changes you need to.

Whatever is stopping you, or holding you back from achieving your full potential in life, *exactly the same thing is stopping you from talking to God.*

If you'll say you have no time, I guarantee that's a big problem in every other area of your life, too. If you say you can't see the point of doing it, you'll also have that same attitude in other important areas of your life. If you believe you can't do it, and that you're going to fail if you try - Bingo! Now you know why you're also stuck in so many other areas of your life.

So pay close attention to what's stopping you from working on your GodJuice, because it'll be precisely the same thing that's stopping you from happily living your life to the fullest in many other areas. The good news is that the more effort you make to overcome the 'issue' that's stopping you from talking to God, the more it will start to fade away and stop causing you problems in the rest of your life, too.

Getting started

Before you continue reading, take a few seconds to decide how much time you're willing to commit to boosting your GodJuice every day. It can be as little as five minutes, but the key is *to do it every single day without fail.*

If five minutes sounds too hard, how about one minute? Even just one minute of daily GodJuice can move mountains, spiritually and emotionally.

If even one minute sounds too hard (and it can for a lot more people than you might imagine) - don't give up. Read the book anyway, and maybe by the time you get to the end of it, you'll be inspired to start talking to God. Everyone has their own speed and their own pace of change, and the key is to be honest about where you're really holding.

That said, I still want a commitment from you! How much time are you willing to devote to boosting your GodJuice a day?

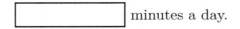 minutes a day.

(One day, you'll thank me for pinning you down on this).

Who's really running the show here?

Another profoundly important reason why consistently working on your GodJuice can change your life, is because it can help you clarify and identify who the 'real you' actually is and it can also help you to see that the 'real you' is genuinely only good.

These days, many of us have no idea which voice in our head is 'the good guy,' and which voice is 'the bad guy.' Is the voice telling me to work overtime 'good' or 'bad'? What about the voice that's telling me to eat some chocolate (purely for health reasons...)? How about the voice that's convinced me I'd be a sucker if I paid my business partner what I really should? I mean, if I pay what I ought to, I'm barely going to have enough to cover my own family's expenses, and surely keeping a roof over my own head has to come ahead of giving some other guy his dues?

It's not always so easy to recognize which voice is 'good' and which voice is 'bad' inside ourselves. A big part of the problem is that our inner bad often dresses itself up as 'good.' It pretends to be our best friend telling us to do these things because it loves us, and it's looking out for us, and it's watching our back.

Then, when it changes back and starts saying that it's only doing that because it's trying to help you, that "you need to know how 'bad' you are, so you can work on it!" your inner bad will screech at you. When it's trying to get you all scared, anxious and upset, it'll start telling you things like: "If you're not aware of the potential issues here, you're going to get yourself in serious trouble!"

When it wants to get you all riled up and furious, it'll start off by telling you something very lofty, like: "There's an important principle at stake here! You're being taken for a ride! What, you're just going to let this jerk step all over you?!? How can *that* be a good thing???"

But of course, all these discussions won't help you at all, and they're actually doing the exact opposite. As a general rule of thumb, the voice of your internal bad will do its best to:

- tear you down

- destroy your confidence and optimism

- criticize and judge you harshly

- try to scare the pants off you and attempt to fill you full of bitterness, despair and self-loathing

Often, under the cover of the highest ideals.

By contrast, the real 'you,' the voice of your internal good, or your soul, will always speak kindly and gently to you. It will always encourage you and give you strength, consistently trying to build you up, even when you've repeatedly fallen down. The 'real you' will soothe and calm you with words of comfort, conciliation and strength, as it reminds you that God is running the world, and that God only does things for your ultimate good.

As you start to work on your GodJuice you should find that it gets easier and easier for you to identify which internal voice is actually talking to you. I know this sounds like a no-brainer - I mean, *duh!* Of course the voice telling you to beat up the granny is *bad!* Yet in practice, all of us are getting duped into listening to the wrong voice, every single day.

I want to share a very simple, but powerful tool with you, that I learned from the internationally-acclaimed spiritual coach Shalom Arush. This tool has often helped me to spot when my inner 'bad' is taking me for a ride.

> *Shalom Arush's rule of thumb*
> *If it's a GOOD thought, it's coming from a GOOD place.*
> *If it's a BAD thought, it's coming from a*
> *BAD place. The 'real you' is your soul.*

Your inner 'bad' is usually directly associated with your body, and its 'animal instinct.' It's the part of you that wants the chocolate cake, that wants its own way all the time, that wants an easy life. But your body, important as it is, is *not* the real you. *The real you is your soul.*

So many people are so used to thinking that their body is the real them that they might find this idea profoundly shocking. Remember that the voice of your soul is always trying to build you up, to encourage you to like yourself, and to fill you up with happiness, confidence and optimism.

The voice of your body is usually doing exactly the opposite: it's criticizing you, pulling you down, scaring you, threatening you, berating you, and making you feel terrible about yourself.

Now can you see why working on your GodJuice is so vital to maintaining your emotional and mental health? GodJuice powers up the real you, i.e., your soul, and strengthens the voice of your internal good.

Without a strong, regular dose of GodJuice, it's very hard for most people to internalize that the angry, jealous, critical little guy they're hearing in their heads 24/7 is not the 'real them.'

That guy is shouting, and ranting and raving, while your soul, the real you, is quietly whispering away that it wants to give, and to love unconditionally, and to help, and to forgive.

Regular GodJuice sessions give your soul the stereo speakers it needs to grab your attention, and make itself heard. It puts your soul back in the driving seat, and forces your body to back down, at least a little.

There is a massive fight going on between these two opposing forces throughout your life, and the more you follow the dictates of your soul - the 'real you' - the more healthy you'll get, in every possible way.

The 'real you' is not your anxiety, fear, anger or hatred - that's just your body talking. The more you talk to God, the more you'll remember that the 'real you' is not just a collection of emotions gone haywire, nor a sum of mere physical and mental problems; the 'real you' is only good. Your body just keeps on tripping you up, stealing your GodJuice, and getting in the way.

Spot the difference

I want to help you catch the voice of your inner 'bad' in action. As you've been reading this, I'm willing to bet that you've had a small voice buzzing in your head, whispering to you that 'the real you' is bad, lazy, selfish, etc. It's probably telling you right now that this stuff might apply to other people, (if it's even true...) but it certainly doesn't apply to people as bad, nasty and duplicitous as *you* are.

Know this: that is the voice of your inner 'bad!' It's telling you bad things about yourself, it's coming from a very bad place, and most upsetting of all, it's telling you a whole bunch of whopping big fibs.

Now, let me help you catch the voice of your soul in action. Read the following statements through slowly, and then try to identify the part of yourself that agrees with them:

- God loves me unconditionally.

- God is very happy with me, exactly as I am.

- God only does things to fix me, not to punish me.

- God wants me to be happy, and to love myself exactly as I am.

The part that's happily nodding in agreement with all this stuff is the 'real you.'

Good thoughts = good place

While I was writing this chapter, I had a really bad day. I'd had a nightmare the previous night that really swept the emotional rug from under my feet, and as the day progressed, I started to feel more and more negative, scared and sour.

Usually, I do my energy exercises every morning to get myself going; that day - I couldn't be bothered. Normally, after I spend an hour talking to God, I also try to spend a bit of time saying 'thanks' for random things. That day I felt so far away from God, I couldn't muster up the energy to thank Him for anything.

My hour of GodJuice helped me to actually get out of bed (which shouldn't be underestimated!), but I was still walking around under a huge dark cloud of pessimism, self-pity and anxiety.

My head was filled with thoughts like: "Your book's dumb, no one's interested in anything you've got to say, you're a failure, and you probably always will be."

On the one hand, of course I *knew* it was my inner 'bad' telling me all this stuff, but on the other, it still sounded so plausible and true! Maybe my book really is dumb...maybe I really am a failure...maybe it's all just a huge waste of time after all...

As I was drifting lower and lower, I suddenly remembered what I'd just been working on in this chapter, namely that good thoughts are coming from a good place, and bad thoughts are coming from a bad place.

That thought hit me with a jolt, and I suddenly got a bit of energy to fight back against all the negative energy and emotions swirling around my brain. Once I had clarity that BAD THOUGHTS ONLY COME FROM A BAD PLACE, I gave myself permission to not believe all that internal negative propaganda anymore, and to start to argue back.

Within half an hour, my mood had lifted, although I was still feeling pretty tired and frazzled. But the whole episode showed me once again how powerful and effective the tools and advice in this book really are.

RECAP

A daily dose of GodJuice works on a number of levels; spiritually, emotionally and physically, to:

■ Reduce and eliminate stress.

■ Give you a sense of well-being that radiates out into your body.

■ Give you the spiritual strength and courage to become the 'real you,' and to start doing the things that are physically and mentally good for you, like eating healthier, exercising more, and doing more of the things that make you feel genuinely happy.

■ Help you work out the hints God is sending you about what you might need to work on, change or fix.

■ Enable you to really start seeing God's hand in your life.

■ Help you clarify when the voice of your 'inner good,' or your soul, is talking to you, and when you're listening to your 'inner bad.'

Chapter 3

Be Kind to Yourself: Healthy Compassion

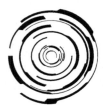

Once you've got your GodJuice back up to strength and humming along, it's time to tackle the next thing that could be closing your body's energy down, and making you sick: bad emotional health habits.

Why your emotions hold the key to your health

These days, every emotion except 'fake happy' seems to have gone out of fashion. You're allowed to be stressed, you're sometimes allowed to be angry (especially at terrorists and 'injustice') and you can cry when your family pet bites the dust - but that's about it.

Today, society is so scared of emotions, particularly negative emotions, that you get hustled straight onto medication if you even show the smallest sign of deviating from 'fake happy.'

In theory, you can see how it kind of makes sense: I mean, no one actually enjoys feeling sad, or lonely, or worthless, or anxious. If there's a fast, effective way of switching those feelings off, why suffer?

There's just one problem with this view: it's complete baloney.

Spiritually, God is sending you your feelings and emotions, even your negative ones, for a good reason. Each time you get sad, frustrated, hurt or depressed, that emotion actually contains a big clue about what you might need to work on, change or fix to start living the happy, healthy, fulfilled life that God has planned for you.

Emotionally, your feelings represent your true self; the 'inner you.' If you try to turn your emotions off and disconnect from the 'real you,' you could end up really struggling to fulfill your potential in life, develop genuine, authentic relationships with other people and feel happy and content - even if you're externally very successful and apparently 'have it all.'

Your feelings don't just magically disappear because you're taking medication. All the meds do is break that connection between your conscious awareness of what you're truly feeling, and the feeling itself.

To put it another way, it's like when the gas light starts flashing on your dashboard. That's a sign that you need to stop at the next gas station, and refill your tank. That little light is actually saving you a huge amount of stress and trouble further on down the road. It's giving you plenty of warning to do what you need to do to replenish your fuel, so you don't get stranded by the side of the road in the middle of nowhere.

Your negative emotions do the same thing. When you get angry, or sad, or critical, it's a warning light that you have habits or behaviors or beliefs that are hurting you, not helping you. You can switch the light off - and many people do - but the underlying problem won't go away.

Let's use anger as an example. If you don't deal with the underlying cause of your anger, your feeling of anger then backs up in your energy system (often, directly affecting the Gallbladder Meridian) - and before you know it, you're experiencing sciatica (excruciating shooting pains down your legs), migraine headaches or you'll start grinding your teeth in your sleep.

The problem can still be fixed at this stage, just like a car can still be filled up with gas even when it's broken down in the middle of nowhere - but it's definitely going to take more time and effort to get the show back on the road.

How to deal with emotions in a healthy way

God gave you your negative emotions, and they're actually meant to serve a useful purpose, once you know how to relate to them and deal with them, in a healthy way.

The ancient Jewish mystical tradition called the Kabbalah explains that your emotions are the connective material between your soul and your body; they connect how you *think* to how you really *feel*. To put it another way, your emotions are the principal route that your subconscious uses to communicate with your intellect (that part of your thought process you have actually some direct control over).

Let's go back to the anger example, to see how this could work in practice. Say you have a friend who routinely makes you feel angry. Maybe they show up at your house unannounced at all times of the day, or they often put you down and embarrass you in front of your peers, or they're very untrustworthy and they frequently make promises they don't stick to.

When someone routinely treats you in a less than caring, disrespectful manner, you usually start feeling pretty angry about that. If you've trained yourself to just tuck your feeling of anger away, and to continue to pretend that everything's fine, even when it really isn't, you are missing the message that God has hidden in your negative emotion.

The message will be different for each of us, but maybe it could be something along the lines of:

- You need to strengthen your boundaries, to make sure people aren't taking advantage of you.

- You need to challenge your friend about their behavior (which will be very hard for you to do, if you hate conflict).

- You need to look inwards, and work out why this particular friend always makes you feel so guilty or sorry for them, that you end up letting them off the hook and excusing their bad behavior.

God will make sure you get exactly the message you need, to begin the next stage of your process of growth and development. When you start paying attention to your negative emotions, you'll learn some amazing things about yourself and why you react to certain people and situations the way you do.

In nearly every circumstance, your negative emotion is coming to tell you that one of the following three areas is out of balance:

- Healthy compassion

- Sensible accountability

- Appropriate kindness

Together, these three things are the foundation of good emotional health. If they're balanced, you'll feel great. If one of them gets out of balance - and in today's world, that can happen all too easily - the repercussions on your physical health and emotional well-being can be tremendous.

Over the coming pages, you're going to learn about each of these foundations in turn, and you'll discover why imbalances in these three areas can affect your health so fundamentally at every level, and what you can do to get back into emotional equilibrium.

The First Foundation of Good Emotional Health: Healthy Compassion

There are two main ways that compassion can get out of balance and unhealthy, in every sense of the word. At one extreme, unhealthy compassion can mean that you're often trying to do everything for everyone else, getting trodden-on in the process, and not taking the time to nurture yourself and to give yourself what you really need. You don't need a PhD in holistic healing to see that if this state of affairs continues for any length of time, it can severely affect your mental, emotional and physical health.

At the other extreme, if you tend to ONLY think about yourself and what you need, and you often act like a selfish jerk who can't 'see' anyone else in the picture, that can also seriously impact your health (and leave you with no friends...).

So how can you strike the balance between these two extremes, and develop spiritually healthy compassion that lets you empathize with other people without getting buried underneath all their problems, or being taken for a ride, or being treated like dirt?

Before I answer that question, let me ask you another one:

Q: When someone is acting in a compassionate way, what does that mean in practice?

- What do they say?

- What do they do?

- How do they act?

- What vibes do they give off?

- How does the other person feel after their interaction?

(You might want to write down your own ideas, before reading on).

When someone has a healthy, balanced sense of compassion then they will:

- Forgive other people easily.

- Forgive themselves easily.

- Try their best not to hold grudges.

- Try their best to avoid dredging up the past.

- Understand that everyone makes mistakes or is occasionally thoughtless.

- Try not to criticize others.

- Try not to blame others (including themselves).

- Care about the other person, their feelings and their experiences.

- Acknowledge, respect and validate their own feelings and needs.

- Really want to help other people (and not just make a lot of noise about doing things for others, which never materializes into actual help).

- Act generously.

- Respect other people, even if they are very different.

- Not insist on 'getting their dues.'

- See the other person's difficulties, issues, or limitations, without making excuses for them, or enabling their negative behavior.

- Not act in an overly-strict or demanding manner with other people.

■ Try to put themselves in the other person's shoes, and to see things from their perspective.

Is there anything else you want to add to this list?

Compassion is NOT the norm today

As you're probably already starting to work out for yourself, healthy compassion is pretty rare in our modern world. When people upset us, inconvenience us, fail to do exactly what we want or what suits us, or damage our possessions in some way, the common response is to get upset and to bite their heads off.

That's the normal way of today's world, but it's not the spiritually healthy way. You could sum up the spiritually healthy way with one word: **empathy**.

The dictionary definition of 'empathy'

My dictionary defines empathy like this: ***the power of entering into another's personality and imaginatively experiencing his experiences.*** Or to put it another way, it's the ability to actually see something from another person's point of view.

If you can't empathize with another person, you'll find it very difficult to treat them compassionately.

Feel yourself, first

If you're starting to realize that you're finding it hard to treat other people with genuine empathy and compassion, don't panic! It's usually only because you haven't experienced very much of it in your own life.

Remember what you learned a little earlier on: compassion is NOT the norm these days, which means that most of us have no idea about how different our lives would be if we were regularly getting more healthy compassion from others.

One of the main aims of this book is to help you to really engage with your feelings and to get back in touch with the 'real you.' Once you're back in touch with the real you, you'll find it much easier to treat others with more compassion and empathy.

But first, let's try to build up a picture of what 'empathy' actually looks like, in real time, by thinking about the following questions:

- How do people act, when they are genuinely empathizing with you?

- What do they do?

- What do they say?

- How do you feel, after you've been 'empathized with'? (This one is crucial...)

When someone is really trying to empathize with you, they'll be genuinely interested in what you're telling them, and they'll show that by asking you pertinent questions about the difficulty, issue or upset you're experiencing. Then when you start speaking, they'll make an effort to really listen to what you're telling them.

If you make it clear that you don't want to talk about it, they'll respectfully back off. If it's obvious you need reassurance, encouragement, or moral support, an empathetic person will do their best to try to reflect those things back at you.

Genuine empathy always contains the following elements:

1. They **ask** about you and / or your situation, and they really want to know what's going on with you.

2. They **listen** attentively to your response.

3. They **reflect** what you're saying, or what you need, back at you.

If you want space, they give you space. If you want reassurance or a shoulder to cry on, a genuinely empathetic person will pick up on your signals and do their best to give you what you need.

But when someone can't truly empathize with you, they'll usually find it next to impossible to treat you compassionately. The following real-life examples shows how this dynamic can play out:

Some Examples of a Lack of Empathy

The Nagging Wife

Mr. Jones has a demanding job, and a rush hour commute of between an hour and an hour and a half, depending on the traffic. He comes home exhausted. Mrs. Jones has no idea how tiring her husband's day is, as she hasn't yet learned to put herself into her husband's shoes, and to empathize with him. As soon as he steps in through the door, she assails him with complaints about her tough day, demands for more help with the chores, and asks him to immediately go upstairs and replace the light bulb that burnt out in the utility room.

Once Mrs. Jones switches into 'compassionate mode,' she'll let her husband unwind a little, and decompress from his day, and maybe even ask him how he's doing, before asking him to take out the garbage.

The Demanding Parent

When Rachel Green's eight-year-old daughter forgot to do her math homework and got a note home from the teacher, her mother hit the roof and started accusing her daughter of all sorts of horrible things. Because Rachel is struggling to empathize with her daughter, she forgot that even adults sometimes forget to do things, particularly things they don't really want to do.

As Rachel starts working on building her sense of empathy, it'll get much easier for her to remember that she also sometimes makes mistakes (like the time she forgot to make the meal for the neighbor like she said she was going to do), which will make it much easier for her to treat her daughter more compassionately.

The Unsympathetic Friend

Esther is one of life's 'winners': she lives in the nicest house, on the best street. She makes the best food, she dresses expensively, she drives the fanciest car, and her husband makes the most money of anyone in the neighborhood. Esther finds it impossible to empathize when her friends are experiencing financial difficulties. As a result, whenever the conversation turns to a difficult money issue her friend is experiencing, Esther either tries to:

- change the subject
- one-up her friend, by telling her about someone else's even harder financial circumstances
- blame her friend for creating her own difficulties
- close the conversation down, with platitudes like 'I'm sure it will all turn out OK.'

Once Esther realizes a more compassionate response is required, she'll give her friends space to share their true feelings, she won't blame them for their problems, and she won't feel like she has to 'fix' everyone else's life.

Don't panic if any of these sound like you! Even the most spiritually healthy person in the world occasionally makes mistakes, and sometimes responds to others with a lack of empathy. Remember that a lack of empathy is the <u>normal</u> response in today's world - and it's a key reason why so many of us feel so anxious and 'off kilter' so much of the time.

As a general rule, when people empathize with you, you *feel* loved, cherished, supported, cared for and safe. When people start blaming you, or criticizing you for your problems, you generally *feel* defensive, angry, 'bad,' worthless, and very lonely. The more you tune into your feelings, the more you'll start to see who's really treating you compassionately, and who isn't.

The Modern Epidemic of Verbal Cruelty

Even though most people generally accept that hitting people or torturing kittens is bad, many people are still very resistant to the idea that using words to hurt people is cruel, or even wrong.

But we usually remember, and suffer from, an unpleasant verbal encounter for much longer than we would a minor physical hardship or injury. Yes, it hurt a lot when I nearly cut the top of my finger off when I was making a salad and I had to get it stitched back together, but once it healed I completely forgot all about it.

By contrast, every time I think of that horrible teacher who made me stand on my chair in front of the whole class while they berated me for being late, I still cringe. Mentally, I'm still suffering from that teacher's cruel speech, and long-term, it's affecting me far more than my damaged finger.

The plain fact is that verbal cruelty can seriously damage your psyche and soul, but it's such a 'normal' occurrence that we normally don't even register what's going on, or how we're physiologically reacting to being mocked, criticized or blamed. The prevalence of cruel speech and behavior in today's world is a key reason why so many people feel so anxious so much of the time, particularly in relation to their social standing and interactions with other people.

Let's define what 'verbal cruelty' actually is. It can take the form of:

- Slurs on your character or reputation

- Offensive, disrespectful speech

- Destructive, demoralizing statements

- Manipulating others; making them feel bad

- Counterproductive and unconstructive comments

- Parodying someone

- Spreading secrets

- Misinforming and misleading people

- Making negative statements in a subtle 'passive-aggressive' way

- Using facial expressions and gestures to put someone else down

The basic rule of thumb is this:

> *Compassionate responses make people feel loved,*
> *cared for and great;*
> *Cruel responses make people feel defensive,*
> *lonely, anxious and angry.*

The following example shows how this could play out in real life:

Example: Family Comes First

After years of barely making ends meet financially, Jake decided he had to leave the family firm, to try and start up his own business. It was a very hard decision for Jake, and he only took it after intense discussions with his wife, who was cracking under the strain of trying - and sometimes failing - to cover the family's most basic expenses.

Jake went to discuss the issue with his brother, and received a very cold reception. His brother appeared to not hear, or to not care, about the extremely difficult circumstances Jake and his family had been struggling with for years.

Every time Jake tried to explain the extreme strain the lack of money was placing on his marriage, his happiness and now also his health, his brother shut him down with platitudes about 'family loyalty' and 'making sacrifices for Dad.' "Our family's always cared more about people than about money," Jake's brother told him, with an arch look that spoke volumes.

Jake left his brother feeling like a disloyal loser and moral failure who was greedy and selfish. In one short conversation, Jake's brother had dismissed all of his years of self-sacrifice, his striving to do the right thing, and his own upset at having to choose between his marriage and staying in the family business. Jake felt completely broken and alone.

Meanwhile, Jake's brother was patting himself on the back for putting Jake back in his place, convinced he'd just acted in the most correct manner possible. Let his brother get his priorities right! Nothing comes before family loyalty, not even Jake's marriage.

The default option

Your default option is to treat others the way you yourself were treated. If you didn't experience a lot of healthy compassion and empathy when you were growing up, you'll probably find it very hard to treat others with compassion (until you learn how to do it). And the people you'll have the least time and consideration for will be:

1. Yourself

2. Your spouse

3. Your kids

The good news is that God can solve any problem. If a lack of compassion for yourself and others is coming up as an issue for you (and once again, let me reassure you that these days, it's an issue for almost everyone) - start talking to talk God about it, and ask Him to help you fix it.

Criticism is also devastating for adults

While I was in the middle of writing this chapter, I had to take my daughter for some tutoring. The tutor lived in a newly-built section of town that didn't appear on my map, and she gave me terrible directions and the wrong street name.

The first time, I got completely lost, and arrived at the tutor's house pretty late. I hate being late, and I was relieved that she was relatively understanding. The second time, I set out in plenty of time to make our appointment - and got stuck in a massive traffic jam right outside my house. I got to my appointment 15 minutes late - and this time, she let me have it with both barrels before I could even open my mouth.

I was ruining everything... she couldn't do anything like this... I may as well not bother if this is how it was going to be... on and on she went. The woman was being paid for her time, regardless of how late we showed up. The problem was ours, not hers, if the lesson wasn't achieving much.

My daughter went in for the rest of her lesson and as soon as the door closed behind her, I burst into tears. I felt so humiliated and inadequate.

Even though I knew what I was dealing with and even though I'm a grown-up, the whole experience was still pretty traumatic and unpleasant, and it really brought home to me, once again, the devastating impact of verbal cruelty.

Getting sensitized to compassionate versus cruel responses

Most people don't react cruelly on purpose; they simply never realized that there was a better, more compassionate way of handling their interactions.

The following scenarios will help you to catch the differences between a compassionate response and a cruel one.

After you read the scenarios, take a couple of minutes to imagine how something similar might be playing out in your own life. What words are popping into your head? What phrases are you using or hearing? How does your body language look? What expression is on your face?

When you're reading the scenarios, try to put yourself in both people's shoes, and pay attention to how you would really *feel*, in these situations.

Scenario 1: The Friend Whose Husband Made a Bad Business Investment, and Went Bankrupt

Jenny's husband, Stewart, has always been a bit of a maverick. Stewart likes to stand out from the crowd, and often comes across as a little idiosyncratic. He's a very smart, charismatic man, and he's not afraid to speak his mind. Many of Stewart's friends have a love / hate relationship with him: they love his flair, colorful opinions and generosity of spirit, but many of them are also more than a little jealous of his accomplishments and apparent financial acumen and success. Jenny, his wife, tends to stay in the background, out of the way, and to just let her larger-than-life husband get on with it.

Recently, one of Stewart's business investments unexpectedly turned sour, leaving the family with a very big hole in their bank balance and a forced sale of their home. Jenny is struggling to find her place in the financial reality, and is frequently feeling overwhelmed and miserable about her current situation. At the same time, she feels fiercely loyal to her husband, and doesn't want to get pulled into any blame games or criticism about what just happened.

Jenny bumps into her friend Suzanne in the local mall, a couple of days after the news of Stewart's business difficulties had started to filter out.

<u>How is the compassionate friend Suzanne going to react to Jenny?</u>

Let's remember the three principles of practical empathy:

1) The Compassionate Friend Asks About You And / Or Your Situation, And They Really Want To Know.

Suzanne the compassionate friend is going to ask Jenny how she's doing, and she's going to be prepared to give her friend some time and her full attention and caring, when she responds. Suzanne realizes that this is not going to be a one minute conversation in between tracking down a bargain at Target and meeting her mom for lunch in the food hall.

2) The Compassionate Friend Listens Attentively To Your Response.

Suzanne the compassionate friend doesn't butt-in with 'quick fixes' or ideas for how to turn everything around, or platitudes. There's a time for brain-storming solutions, and for coming up with practical suggestions for solving a problem, but this isn't it. First, Suzanne is going to give her friend the opportunity to unburden herself to a sympathetic ear. If Jenny doesn't feel like talking about it, she'll respect that - and not continue to fish for more information - and let her friend know that she's there for her in whichever way she can be.

3) The Compassionate Friend Reflects What You Need Back At You.

If Jenny needs encouragement, Suzanne the compassionate friend is going to try to give it to her. If she needs hope, comfort or reassurance, Suzanne the compassionate friend will try to bolster her belief that God can do anything, and can turn it all around.

If Jenny needs understanding - it's so hard to make ends meet now, and Jenny was used to buying whatever she wanted, whenever she wanted it - Suzanne the compassionate friend won't condescend her. She'll give her a hug, and tell her about her own tough patch, and how she got through it and came out much stronger, and that it really is going to be OK. It's definitely a big test, but God never gives people tests that are bigger than they are.

Jenny comes away from the meeting with Suzanne her compassionate friend feeling a tad more reassured, a drop more optimistic that everything is going to turn out OK, and a whole lot less lonely.

Now, let's flip the coin and see:

How would Suzanne the cruel friend act?

Suzanne the cruel friend either doesn't want to know what's going on with Jenny her bankrupt buddy, OR will relish hearing all the gritty details, even if Jenny doesn't want to discuss them (especially not in the middle of the mall, where anyone can hear them).

If Suzanne the cruel friend is the prying type, she'll ask probing, insensitive questions like: "How are your kids coping with all this?" Or: "How are you going to fit all your gorgeous furniture into a tiny apartment? You're probably going to have to sell your antique dining set, too." Or, she'll tell Jenny that housing is going really cheap in some low-rent area that no one from their circle would ever dream of living in.

If Suzanne is the dismissive type, then she'll hear Jenny out in stony-cold silence. There'll be no condolences, no sympathy, and no encouragement. At some point, Suzanne the cruel friend will start to get bored with what she feels is Jenny's whining and self-pity, and will decide to shut her friend up by telling her that everyone knew that it was a dumb investment, and that she only has herself to blame for not reining Stewart in.

If Suzanne the cruel friend is having a good day, she'll offer Jenny a rather flat 'there, there,' pat her friend's arm insincerely, and then start excitedly discussing her own plans to upgrade her kitchen.

Jenny will come away from her meeting with Suzanne, the cruel friend, feeling demoralized, patronized, despairing, angry and very, very alone.

Scenario 2: The Big Boss

David has a serious job, with a serious law firm. Deadlines are set in stone, with staff regularly expected to work through the night to complete a deal. All 'i's' must be dotted, all 't's' must be crossed. The firm's reputation is at stake.

David usually loves the cut and thrust of being a successful corporate lawyer, but one afternoon in the middle of doing yet another 'big deal,' he gets a phone call to tell him his father has just unexpectedly died from a heart attack.

How is Barry, David's boss and senior partner on the 'big deal,' going to react now that his main man has been taken out of action?

How is the compassionate boss Barry going to react to David's news?

1) The Compassionate Boss Asks About You And / Or Your Situation, And Really Wants To Know.

Barry knows that David was close to his father. As soon as he finds out the news, he calls David into his office to ask him what the funeral arrangements are and how much time off David will need to really come to terms with the tragic and sudden loss of his father.

David is struggling to hold it together emotionally, but he is also worried about 'letting the side down' on the deal, which he knows is really important to Barry. He's unsure of what to do - try to complete the deal, and then leave in a few hours, or leave now but cause big problems for Barry...

2) The Compassionate Boss Listens Attentively To Your Response.

Barry immediately picks up that the only thing keeping David in the office right now is his sense of loyalty to Barry.

3) The Compassionate Boss Reflects What You Need Back At You.

Barry takes control of the situation, and insists that David get his things together, and go do whatever he needs to do - and that he should take as much time off as he needs, to really mourn his father properly.

Barry takes great pains to reassure David that they've got it all covered, and that he'll just pull in a few junior partners to finish off the loose ends of the deal.

"Turn your phone off, and keep it off for at least a week," he tells David. "These things hit us very hard, and you need to go and be with your family. The last thing I want you to be doing is checking your emails or worrying about this deal. We have it all covered, and if something unexpected crops up, we'll deal with it."

David feels reassured, comforted and much less stressed by his boss's compassionate reaction, which took all the pressure of the deal off his shoulders, enabling him to properly manage a very shocking and tragic situation.

Now, let's see how Barry the cruel boss would have reacted:

Barry is furious at David for putting additional pressure on him in the middle of the deal, and he's not trying to hide it.

He knows, technically, that David couldn't help his father having a heart attack at such an inconvenient time, but that doesn't stop him from sniping at David and criticizing him for leaving far too much of the deal 'to the last minute,' now leaving him, Barry, with 'a huge mess.'

Barry isn't interested in what happened or how David feels about it. He just wants to know two things: "What's the latest you can leave here, and still make it to the funeral?" And then, "How soon can you get back to the office?"

Barry is furious, frustrated, and mega-stressed, barking orders at David left right and center. Every time David starts trying to get his stuff together to leave, Barry waylays him with another last-minute concern. As David gets increasingly agitated about being delayed in the office - he's getting a lot of distressed calls from his newly-widowed mother and siblings, and he can't really talk to them - Barry goes ballistic, and starts berating him loudly in front of his colleagues, for being 'sloppy,' and 'cavalier,' and a bad lawyer.

Barry is completely oblivious to the huge emotional explosion that's just occurred in David's life, and can only see himself, and his own stress and frustrations.

As David is finally making it out through the door, Barry barks one last order at him: "Keep your phone on at all times! If I need some info, I want you to be able to give it to me, even if they're still shoveling the dirt!"

David is thunderstruck, and leaves feeling conflicted, worried, stressed and incredibly tense about the coming few days. How is he going to manage if Barry calls in the middle of his father's eulogy? His mother would never forgive him for taking the call...

Scenario 3: The Dead Pet

After months of nagging, Emma finally gave in, and bought her 10-year-old daughter a budgie. Emma laid down some clear rules right from the start: the pet was her daughter's responsibility, and she was responsible for cleaning the cage and making sure the budgie had enough food and drink.

Emma's daughter was over the moon with her new pet, but Emma was less thrilled. It made a lot of noise, it made a lot of mess, and when her daughter forgot to clean the cage out, it could really stink.

One week, the budgie started to look very fat, and couldn't seem to stop eating. It was pecking away at everything, including the pretty napkin her daughter had put on the bottom of the cage to decorate it.

Emma suddenly realized that the napkin had got stuck in the bird's digestive system, and that the budgie was trying to dislodge the block by eating everything in sight. With the insight of a grown-up, Emma realized her daughter's pet didn't have much longer to live.

The next day, her daughter came to her half-hysterical: the budgie had died.

How is Emma the compassionate parent going to react?

1) The Compassionate Parent Asks How Their Child Is Feeling, And They Really Want To Know.

Emma goes to check that the budgie is really dead - it's true. As she confirms it, her daughter bursts into tears and starts sobbing.

Emma puts an arm around her child, and hugs her. Her daughter starts to beat herself up: maybe she didn't give the bird enough food, or change the water often enough, or clean out the cage properly (all of which might be true...).

2) The Compassionate Parent Listens Attentively To Their Child's Response.

Emma realizes that her daughter is feeling guilty and somehow 'to blame' for the bird's death. She reassures her daughter that she looked after her pet superbly, and gave it the best possible care and attention. It was just the bird's time, that's all.

Her daughter stops crying, but still looks very upset and still has the nagging guilt that "maybe I didn't look after it properly?"

3) The Compassionate Parent Reflects Back At Their Child What They Really Need.

Emma patiently reassures her daughter that she gave her pet 5-star care and attention. It's not her fault the bird died; God decided it was time, and that's all. She continues to hug her daughter, and then asks her daughter what sort of 'burial' she'd like to give her pet.

The daughter is still sad, but feels cared for, sympathized with, and reassured that she isn't to blame for her bird dying.

How is the cruel parent Emma going to react?

(Before you read on, let me re-emphasize that you can only have healthy compassion for your children if you first have healthy compassion for yourself. We'll come back to this topic in much greater detail later on.)

Emma hears the bird has died, and has this overwhelming impulse to tell her traumatized daughter what she must have done wrong to cause it:

"It's that napkin you put into the cage!! The bird ate it, and it stuffed up its stomach. Why didn't you ask me before you did that??"

Her daughter is terror-struck, her worst fear just got confirmed: she *is* to blame for her pet dying. She feels absolutely terrible, like the worst person in the world.

Emma is oblivious to the emotional tsunami that's just swept her daughter away, and is already bustling into the bedroom, and disposing of the budgie; straight into a plastic bag, then into the garbage and from there, straight out of the house. Dead birds are very unclean things.

Her daughter watches all this in stunned silence, but Emma doesn't notice. She's pleased as punch that the 'problem pet,' with its 'problem food' has disappeared out of her life, and she couldn't be happier about it.

"Cheer up!" she tells her miserable-looking daughter. "At least now, I don't have to keep vacuuming the carpet in your room every day!"

HOW UNHEALTHY COMPASSION CAN AFFECT YOUR HEALTH

Unhealthy compassion can affect your emotional and mental health in the following ways:

SPIRITUALLY: It can disconnect you from God.

EMOTIONALLY:

1) When you spend a lot of time around people with limited compassion and empathy, it can make you feel:

- uncared for

- unloved

- unsupported

- disrespected, and even

- worthless.

In turn, this can cause you to react with a strong negative emotion like:

- Anger

- Fear

- Anxiety

- Vengeance

- Jealousy (of other people who appear to be getting more compassion and caring)

2) When you're not treating others with enough healthy compassion

If you typically haven't been treating other people with as much compassion as you could have (and again, join the club, because healthy compassion is NOT the norm today) - then you usually end up feeling pretty bad about yourself, afterwards.

This can lead to you experiencing chronic feelings of guilt, self-hatred and shame, which can be even more painful and damaging to you, long-term, than a physical injury or trauma.

PHYSICALLY: A lack of compassion can keep you feeling wound-up and permanently stressed out, which has obvious implications for your physical health.

The good news is that it's fairly easy to fix unbalanced compassion when you've got God on board and you've already recognized the problem.

You'll find practical ideas and solutions for how you can get your compassion back into healthy, balanced mode in the second half of the book.

RECAP

- Emotionally unhealthy habits can seriously affect your mental, emotional and physical health.

- The three foundations of good emotional health are:

  1. **Healthy Compassion**

  2. **Sensible Accountability**

  3. **Appropriate Kindness**

- Healthy compassion means that you are able to see the other person's side of things and able to empathize with their pain, without getting stepped on or taken advantage of.

- The effects of emotional pain, like shame, fear and guilt, are usually much greater, and much longer-lasting than the effects of physical pain.

- Verbal cruelty is the opposite of healthy compassion.

- If you don't have a lot of healthy compassion for yourself and others, perhaps it is because you didn't experience a lot of healthy compassion when you were growing up, and / or your Spleen Meridian energy is very depleted and needs strengthening.

- Healthy compassion is not the norm in today's world, which is one of the main reasons why so many people feel anxious and on edge when dealing with others.

■ To fix deficient compassion we need to:

- Recognize the problem

- Get God involved

- Practice the three rules of responding compassionately to others

- Strengthen our Spleen Meridian energy.

Chapter 4

Sensible Accountability:

When It's Good to Say Sorry

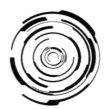

The second foundation of emotional health is sensible accountability. In today's topsy-turvy world, far too many of us are walking around feeling bad for things that we have no control over, and are not feeling ashamed about things that we really should be ashamed of.

So when is it 'healthy' to feel ashamed and accountable? And how can you know if the accountability and shame you're feeling is actually helpful and spiritually-positive, or toxic and spiritually-damaging? This chapter is all about finding some answers to these crucially important questions.

Defining healthy accountability

Before we jump into the whole discussion about what makes accountability healthy, we need to define what accountability actually *is*. For the purposes of this book, the definition of accountability I'm going to use is:

Taking appropriate responsibility for something you did wrong.

In its proper context, accountability (and the feelings of guilt and shame that often prompt it) is a very useful trait to have and a key component of our spiritual makeup or soul.

God gave you (and me, and everyone else out there) the ability to feel accountable and ashamed of our behavior for the following reasons:

- If you never feel ashamed about the things you've done that are objectively wrong, you won't try to make amends for them.

- Shame can motivate you to change and improve.

- When you feel accountable for how you act, and how you treat others, that makes it much more likely that you'll more often relate to people with more kindness and compassion.

When your feelings of accountability motivate you to clean up the mess you made, or to sincerely apologize for something you did wrong, or to resolve to get a grip on your bad character traits, then they're coming from a healthy place, and they're actually doing you a world of good, spiritually, emotionally and physically.

When your feelings of accountability are either completely absent, or are crippling you with feelings of toxic shame and guilt, then that's seriously unhealthy.

How sensible accountability looks, in real time

So let's take a look at how 'sensible accountability' actually appears, in real time.

When a person is emotionally healthy, and their sense of accountability is balanced, they will normally act in the following ways, if they've done something wrong. They will:

- Own up

- Try to make amends

- Feel guilty (more on this in a minute)

■ Act ashamed (their body language will be soft, not aggressive, head bowed, eyes downcast, they'll probably speak softly and hesitantly)

■ Change their behavior

■ Sincerely apologize for their behavior, and ask for forgiveness

That is how emotionally-healthy accountability looks in action, when a person truly feels regret about something they genuinely did wrong and then tries to make amends for what they did, without beating themselves up or getting paralyzed by guilt feelings.

Unhealthy accountability

Now that we've defined sensible accountability, it's time to take a look at how accountability can get unhealthy and unbalanced. Normally, that can happen in one of two main ways. Either:

1. **You don't give a hoot about who your actions are hurting and you don't feel bad about anything you do, even the worst things in the world.**

OR

2. **You take responsibility for everything that's going wrong in the whole world, and you walk around feeling permanently guilty and 'to blame.'**

I'm exaggerating (a little...) to make the point, but you get the idea. Now, let's look at both of these areas in more detail to try to understand a little more about what's actually causing the problem and what you can do to start resolving it.

Nobody does this right all the time

Before you continue reading, you should know that even the most sincere, saintly, altruistic person will occasionally lose their temper; or talk on their phone while they're driving; or take the last chocolate in the box, even though they know their husband would have really liked it.

Developing sensible accountability does NOT depend on you always acting appropriately and properly - if it did, it would be a spiritual Mission Impossible, because none of us are angels, and we all make mistakes. Rather, sensible accountability is much more about ensuring that you react in a healthy, sensible way AFTER your inevitable error of judgment, mistake, or bad behavior.

So the first question to ask yourself is:

> *Do you own up when you make a mistake or act inappropriately, or do you try to shove it under the carpet and pretend it never happened?*

A little later on in the book, I'll give you some tools and exercises you can use to find out.

When is it good to feel bad?

One of the main reasons why you might find it difficult to take responsibility for something you're genuinely doing wrong could be if you were routinely blamed, criticized or shamed about even minor things when you were growing up. If you were off mugging grannies or hijacking cars - well, OK then, that might have been an appropriate response from your caregivers.

But if you were just making honest mistakes, or errors of judgment, or acting in an immature way, (which is 100% OK, considering that you were a CHILD) then you might have turned off your ability to feel responsible as a defense mechanism.

(It's timely to note here that your caregivers were probably raised with the same sort of parenting paradigm they handed on to you. They were doing the best they could, given that no one was talking about healthy compassion and sensible accountability 50 years ago.)

The good news is that just as your sense of accountability got switched off or numbed, it can get reactivated again. The first step is to identify when it really is 'good' to feel 'bad,' and what you genuinely do need to take responsibility for.

There's so much political correctness and social conditioning permeating the atmosphere these days, that it's really difficult to know what's right and what's wrong. Should you feel terrible if you wiped your mouth on the tablecloth? What about if you yelled at your kid for coming home late? Was it OK that you didn't stand up and give your seat to the old lady on the bus, because you actually felt pretty weak and poorly yourself?

How can you know what you really need to be working on, and what's actually not such a big deal?

This is a big question, and it requires a clear answer, because you can only use shame in the spiritually-healthy way that God intended if you first find an objective and universal benchmark for human behavior that makes it clear what's GOOD and what's BAD - and the good news is, that such a thing exists: it's called the 10 Commandments.

You might want to take a moment to Google the 10 Commandments, (or even, to go and look them up the old-fashioned way) before you continue reading, to remind yourself of what they actually say.

For the purposes of this particular discussion, I've pulled out the essential points of the 10 Commandments, and made them even easier to remember and relate to. If you do any of the following things, what I like to call the five BIG no-no's, then you really should do the following things: you really should feel ashamed of yourself, take responsibility for your bad behavior, and try to fix the mess you made:

The five BIG no-no's

- **You killed someone**

- **You stole something**

- **You abused someone else, verbally or physically**

- **You acted immorally**

- **You lied**

That's it! Unless you're a Mafia kingpin, you should be feeling pretty good about yourself right now. If you think about all of the things that you routinely feel embarrassed or ashamed about (including putting on weight, having bad table manners or not earning a fortune) you'll see that many of the things you're beating yourself up about simply don't fit the above criteria.

You didn't kill anyone... so why do you still feel so guilty?

But what if you *know* you shouldn't feel ashamed about driving your old jalopy around, and you *know* you're not mugging any grannies on the street, but you still feel bad about yourself, and you still feel guilt-ridden and anxious around other people? What's going on with *that?*

The answer is that you need to go back to the first foundation of emotional health, and make strengthening your compassion for yourself one of your main priorities.

When you don't have enough self-compassion that can lead to all sorts of unhealthy emotional habits, including:

- beating yourself up for making honest errors and mistakes

- blaming yourself whenever things go wrong, and

- getting angry with yourself, just for having normal feelings and problems (and not being 'perfect').

In the worst case scenarios, a severe lack of self-compassion can leave you feeling worthless, empty and 'fatally-flawed,' as though you have nothing left to give and no reason to be alive. But no one can be perfect all the time! You're a human being, not an angel, and human beings - even the best ones - make a lot of mistakes.

The middle path to sensible accountability

In the following exercise you're going to learn a powerful tool for balancing your sense of accountability, so you're not busy trying to pretend you're perfect all the time, and you're also not blaming yourself for everything that's going wrong in the world.

Developing a 'Voice of Reason'

The following exercise shows you how to develop your own 'Voice of Reason,' which will help you to start relating to yourself in a kinder, more compassionate and more realistic way. Whenever you sense that your accountability is out of whack - either you're trying to wiggle out of something you should be taking responsibility for, or you're beating yourself up over everyone else's problems - activate the following three rules:

Voice of Reason Rule 1:
Remember Nobody's Perfect, And We All Make Mistakes

Instead of beating yourself up when you make an honest mistake, forgive yourself, and try to learn from the experience. Don't stew over it for days or berate yourself for being a worthless idiot.

I know I've already said this, but it really bears repeating: we all mess up and make mistakes. It's part of the human condition. Only a robot could never make a mistake - but even robots occasionally break down and malfunction, so give yourself a break!

Voice of Reason Rule 2:
Treat Yourself At Least As Nicely As You Treat Other People

Don't let your critical voice say anything to you that you wouldn't say to someone else you care about. If you wouldn't call your friend derogatory names under the same circumstances, then don't say it to yourself, either. The following example makes this point very nicely:

Example: The Parking Problem

Let's say you're 20 minutes late to an appointment because you didn't realize parking would be such an issue. If you wouldn't call your friend 'a moron' for finding it hard to park, and get all het up with them for making that mistake, then please don't it to yourself, either.

Before you start beating yourself up and berating yourself, just take a minute and think how you would encourage a friend of yours who'd found themselves in the same situation. Wouldn't you try to look for the good in the situation? Wouldn't you try to show them how it could have happened to anyone, and that they shouldn't take it so personally? Someone with good spiritual health habits would try to find a way to turn it all around, and to show their friend that it really wasn't the overwhelming problem they believed it to be.

Just as you'd do that for your friend, you can also do that for *yourself*.

Voice of Reason Rule 3:
Don't Go To Extremes - Just Look for the Message

When you grow up, for whatever reason, without having a caring parent's 'Voice of Reason' to help you accept and deal with your mistakes in a positive way, your 'inner bad' immediately steps in to fill the gap with two extreme voices. Either:

1. It uses the harsh, castigating, critical 'you idiot!' voice;

OR

2. It goes with the 'letting-yourself-off-the-hook,' 'don't look at this, in case it makes you feel bad' voice.

The first voice is just beating you up, making you feel bad about yourself, and stealing all of your energy. The second voice is encouraging you to avoid all responsibility for your actions, which makes it much more likely that you're going to end up repeating your mistake or bad behavior again in the future.

Remember, God gave you a sense of accountability to encourage and motivate you to change and improve. When you pointlessly start beating yourself up for being less-than-perfect, or when you go into denial about what you're really doing, you're missing the whole point.

What you should be feeling bad, ashamed and guilty about

If you didn't just deliberately break one of the five BIG no-no's (feel free to check back a couple of pages, to refresh your memory about what they actually are), then you shouldn't be feeling bad, guilty or ashamed of yourself. Period.

Let's be clear that if you didn't just kill someone, steal a car, or run away with the neighbor's spouse, you shouldn't be feeling ashamed of yourself.

And you certainly SHOULDN'T feel ashamed of yourself that:

- You don't come from a family of wealthy blue-bloods

- You had a difficult childhood

- You sometimes feel overwhelmed, or sad, or stressed, or down - these are normal feelings

- You're not as svelte as you used to be

- You aren't a genius

- None of your kids made the honor roll in school

- You break out in hives if you spend more than three hours with certain members of your family

- You're broke

- You burnt the cake

- There are hairballs the size of small mammals in the corner of your dining room

- Your latest business venture just spectacularly failed

- You feel lonely, unlovable and anxious some days

- Your child's still sucking their thumb, and they're 16 already...

It's normal to feel, full stop

Feelings and passions, even negative feelings and passions, are completely NORMAL. The only people who can be superficially 'happy' all the time are the people who are taking mood-altering medications. Everyone else will go through a gamut of emotions every single day, as they react to all the different stimuli being sent their way, both for the good, and for the inevitably bad.

If certain people start telling you that you're over-emotional or over-sensitive because you occasionally cry or look a little glum, or that they're worried you aren't coping properly because you're not 100% switched-on and 'happy' 100% of the time - the chances are very high that THEY are the ones with the real emotional problems.

Emotionally healthy and balanced individuals already know that most negative emotions are not something to run away from, or to be embarrassed and ashamed about. They're just messages from God, and they need to be addressed, decoded and dealt with.

It's normal to feel anxious sometimes

Joan had just moved to a new city, and was feeling a little overwhelmed with all the sudden changes in her life. Her husband had a new job, the kids had new schools, Joan had a new routine, and a whole bunch of 'new' people to meet - and her head was spinning so fast, she didn't know what to do with herself.

As the social invitations started to pour in, Joan's feelings of anxiety increased. Yes, people were being so nice and friendly, but the kids were still very unsettled, and it wasn't easy to keep taking them to strangers for meals, however well-meaning people were being.

The worst was when people just wouldn't take 'no' for an answer, and kept pressuring her to come to their meal / event / bingo evening / charity night / bake sale - all for a good cause!!

Joan started to feel increasingly stressed and 'out of it' and she started to worry that she wasn't going to be able to cope with her new reality.

There was too much going on, and she just couldn't handle it! Maybe her friends were right, and she needed 'something' to help her manage. I mean, *everyone else* was coping just fine with their circumstances. Joan seemed to be the only one who was falling apart, and she started to feel really ashamed of herself, as a result.

Secretly, she started to panic that *there **must** be something wrong with her, for feeling this way...*

When the 'emotional charge' is overwhelming

While the vast majority of negative emotions are nothing to worry about, especially once you know how to deal with them, sometimes, negative emotions have been building up in your subconscious for so long that they start to be debilitating or disturbing.

It's beyond the scope of this book to go into a big discussion of why that might be occurring, but when negative emotions come packaged together with such an overwhelming 'charge,' the root cause is usually a disturbing event, experience or trauma (or series of disturbing experiences) that occurred in childhood.

The adult you probably can't even remember what happened, but part of your subconscious somehow got 'stuck' at that stage, at the age the traumatic experience occurred, and whenever something in your present life triggers that subconscious memory or feeling, you can find yourself dealing with some hugely uncomfortable and overwhelming feelings, without really knowing why you're reacting like that.

These types of overwhelming feelings can be very upsetting emotionally, and can even cause you some notable physical sensations and discomfort. The good news is, as soon as you trace the feeling back to its original cause, and properly address it, your negative symptoms and physical reactions will usually disappear immediately.

There are a variety of tools and techniques you can use to do that. You'll find some of them set out in this book a little later on, and you'll find even more useful links, information, techniques and tools on my website, **www. jemi.website.**

Energy Psychology techniques like the Emotional Freedom Technique (EFT) or Tapas Acupressure Technique (TAT), to name just two of the most popular techniques out there, can help you to defuse overwhelming or highly-charged emotions fast, easily and effectively. If you're experiencing anxiety, panic attacks or any other overwhelming or debilitating emotion, I highly recommend you give some of these Energy Psychology techniques a try, before exploring other therapeutic avenues.

Unresolved childhood traumas aside, let me say it again that:

Emotions... even strong emotions... even strong negative emotions... are completely normal and usually very healthy.

They are just prompts for you to change course, or fix something, or learn something, or do something different.

Unfortunately, these days, lots of people can't handle emotions, even healthy ones. That's why it can often happen that when you're trying to open up to another person, you can hit a wall of apathy, blame or aggression, simply because the other person can't handle what you're trying to share. If that happens to you, don't feel bad or start to blame yourself! Simply change the subject, and find someone else to talk to who isn't scared by strong feelings.

One last time: When is it 'good' to feel 'bad'?

God gives everyone exactly the circumstances they need in order to develop their true potential, and to work on their flaws. Sometimes, that might mean that you have to be poor for a bit, or live in a grotty place, or have a bout of ill health, or experience difficult relationships - and all of this is occurring *through no fault of your own*.

Your successes are a present from God, and so are your failures. Everything that happens to you is just part of some massive Divine plan, and God can turn all the circumstances of your life around in, quite literally, the blink of an eye.

Remember that these days, the hardest tests and the biggest work to be done usually occurs closer to home. In our generation, it's much, much easier to be a CEO of a multi-million dollar start-up than it is to have a good marriage and to raise happy, emotionally healthy kids. History is full of people who made great business deals and loads of money, but who were lousy human beings.

I know that's not how it always looks on Facebook. But if your old friend from high school, who now owns a yacht and has three mansions, had to live in your dingy apartment, with your loud neighbors and your moldy carpet, they'd probably have jumped off a bridge a long time ago - which should actually make you feel great about yourself! Why? Because it underlines just how much sticking power, courage and resilience you have; but unfortunately, those aren't the sort of successes that are easy to boast about on your Facebook page.

The point is, you shouldn't feel ashamed about being poor, socially inept, unemployed, messy, emotional, fat or unable to fix everyone else's problems and issues. The only things you should really feel ashamed about are:

> *Serious, immoral things that you are doing wrong.*

Some examples of real things you should be ashamed about might include:

- Abusing your children

- Killing someone

- Running away with the milkman

At the risk of repeating myself, some examples of things you should DEFINITELY NOT be ashamed about include:

- Failing to meet other people's unreasonable expectations

- Making honest mistakes

- Not being in control of the world

- Being unable to 'fix' other people's problems

- Putting yourself, your spouse and your kids first

Remember: If someone fails to accept that you aren't to blame for things going wrong in your life, or that you have a right to say 'no' (even for no reason), or that it's not your job to try to fix their life, it's usually because *they* have a massive problem.

Hopefully, it should now be 1000% clear that if you didn't just kill someone, steal a car, or run away with the neighbor's spouse, you shouldn't be feeling ashamed of yourself. If you did do one of those things, own up, make amends, and ask God to help you to not do it again. Now, put it behind you, and move on.

HOW UNHEALTHY ACCOUNTABILITY CAN AFFECT YOUR HEALTH

Few things can impact your health more dramatically, or more negatively, than the toxic feelings of shame, guilt and self-loathing that come along with unhealthy accountability. When you consistently feel that you're a 'bad' person, the first place you take the hit is your GodJuice.

SPIRITUALLY: If you keep telling yourself that God couldn't possibly be interested in someone like *you,* your GodJuice can drop through the floor, making it hard for you to even get out of bed in the morning.

EMOTIONALLY: Unhealthy accountability means that you either walk around wracked with guilt all the time, or you just shut down your ability to respond to other people's hurt, suffering and pain - even when it's justified, and even when you're the one who's actually causing it.

While these are two extremes of behavior, they revolve around the same very damaging emotional issue (aka 'toxic shame'), namely:

> *You don't like yourself enough, you don't value yourself enough, and you don't think you'll ever really be good enough.*

This can contribute to the development of the following negative emotions:

- Anger
- Defensiveness
- Aggressiveness
- Insensitivity
- Recklessness
- Over-sensitivity
- Fear (particularly fear of doing something wrong or being punished)
- Guilt
- Anxiety
- Resentment

PHYSICALLY: When you don't like yourself, you carry that feeling around with you 24/7. It's very hard to live with someone you don't like; it's hard to care for them properly, it's hard to see the good in them and it's hard to treat them considerately.

All this can impact your energy meridians in a myriad of ways and cause a number of physical issues. As a broad rule of thumb, unhealthy accountability habits often show up as problems connected to the Spleen, Heart, Liver and Gallbladder Meridians.

We'll explore these connections in much more detail in Chapter 7, when we start to look at the relationship between emotions and physical illnesses in much more depth.

RECAP

- Healthy accountability is when you feel remorse and regret when you've genuinely done something wrong, and you take steps to fix the mess you made.

- God doesn't want you to be ashamed or anxious about how you look, what you've achieved, where you live, who your family is, who you are, how much money you have, how fat you might be, or for not being 'happy' all the time.

- God also doesn't want you to be ashamed of making honest mistakes and errors, or for failing to fix other people's problems and issues.

- Sensible accountability depends on having healthy self-compassion.

- When you judge yourself with the VOICE OF REASON that means you don't beat yourself up, and you don't let yourself off the hook for your bad behavior.

Chapter 5

Appropriate Kindness - But Not What You Might Expect

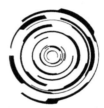

Few things can cause you more anxiety, stress, guilt and self-anger than getting caught up in other people's unhealthy expectations of 'doing good' and the mistaken belief that helping others is ALWAYS a good thing.

The truth is that all sorts of things get packaged up as 'kindnesses,' when they actually aren't. For something to really be a kindness, in the truest sense of the word, it should meet the following four criteria:

1. It has to actually be experienced as a kindness by the recipient

2. It should be 'string-free,' with no expectation of payback

3. You have to really *want* to do it, i.e., it shouldn't feel like an obligation or duty

4. It needs to come from a place of empathy and compassion

When these criteria aren't met, you can get caught up in a spiritually-unhealthy, stress and anxiety-inducing web of expectation, manipulation and obligation, until you recognize some 'kindnesses' are anything but...

That's why 'Appropriate Kindness' is the third, and last foundation of good emotional health. In this chapter, we're going to explore what appropriate kindness actually is; why the four criteria set out above are so important; and why your health can depend upon you being able to tell the difference between true kindnesses and manipulative ploys.

> The first criteria for Appropriate Kindness: The kindness
> has to be experienced as a kindness by the recipient

If the 'help' a person is giving to you is:

- Shaming you

- Embarrassing you

- Belittling you

- Making you feel inferior (by showing the other person's obvious superiority)

- Demeaning you

- Mocking you

- Emasculating you

- Weakening you

- Controlling you

Then it's NOT a true kindness, regardless of how it looks, or how it's being spun.

The following story can hopefully shed a little more light on the subject of why being 'helped' by other people isn't always as 'helpful' or as kind as it initially appears to be:

Example: Rhonda's 'helpful' friend

Rhonda had always been interested in the idea of home-schooling, so she was thrilled to meet Anna, the undisputed Queen of home-schooling who'd educated all five of her children herself, when she moved into their neighborhood. The two hit it off really well, and Rhonda eagerly lapped up all the advice, tips and knowledge Anna was only too happy to share with her.

After a couple of months, Rhonda decided that she wanted to explore the option of home-schooling her own children next term, and she eagerly engaged Anna in the process of helping her to find the right home-schooling resources and framework for her family.

Initially, Anna was quite helpful and made all the right noises, but as it became obvious that Rhonda was serious about home-schooling, Anna's 'helpful advice' became less and less helpful. Anna knew that Rhonda really respected her opinion, and she made no bones about shooting down every single idea or proposal that Rhonda presented to her: this home-schooling program was too faddy, that one had a bad reputation, this one was low-quality, that one was high-quality but too intellectually-demanding for Rhonda's family...

All of Anna's 'helpful advice' left Rhonda feeling very disillusioned and confused about which home-schooling program to participate in, so in the end, she decided to shelve the whole idea.

In the end, Anna's kindness and 'help' ended up being anything but.

How does the kindness feel?

In this chapter, we're going to start digging underneath the external, tangible layer of kindness to see what's really going on. It's not enough to know that your Aunty Gayle sent you a sweater for your birthday, because the true gauge of kindness is how it actually *felt* to receive it.

Did you feel loved and cared for, when you received the kindness, or did you feel mugged, degraded and bad about yourself, in some way? When people are treating you with compassion and empathy - when they really want to help you, without any vested interests - you can really feel it.

A few months prior to starting this book, I got into my first ever, serious car crash. Thank God, no one suffered even so much as a scratch, despite the fact that I had a very elderly woman in my car, and I crashed into a vehicle full of small children. But even with all the miracles God did for me, it was still a challenging time, not least because my car insurance had accidentally lapsed, leaving me to pay for the hefty damage done to the other vehicle out of my own pocket.

My finances were going through a pretty tight time anyway, so I had to swallow my pride, and accept any help that was offered to me. It was not a fun experience, but it was worth its weight in gold, because it ended up teaching me some invaluable lessons about the true nature of kindnesses, which I'd like to share with you.

Keep the cash

When one person offered me a small gift of money, I started sobbing uncontrollably. My reaction took both her and me by surprise, and I couldn't understand why I found it so hard to accept her offer. It's not like she was asking me to sell a kidney in order to pay my rent, or something. Afterwards, I realized that the *way* this person offered me the money made me feel incredibly demeaned and ashamed. Once I realized how much that person was looking down on me, I decided I wasn't going to accept any more 'kindnesses' from that particular individual.

On a different occasion, another person showed up at my front door with boxes and boxes of food, and strangely, I wasn't embarrassed or upset at all. I just felt loved, understood and cared for - and again, my reaction took me completely by surprise. Until that point, I thought getting care packages from my friends would be completely mortifying, and akin to being in purgatory!

The point here is that while many 'kindnesses' can look identical from the outside, the way the kindness is being done, and the place it's coming from can make all the difference to how it's actually being experienced. It's not just about how it looks, it's much more about how it really feels, and that's a crucial distinction.

> ### The second criteria for Appropriate Kindness:
> ### The kindness has to be string-free

Many of our normal interactions with other people are usually based on the principle of mutual benefit, aka 'you scratch my back, and I'll scratch yours.' There's nothing wrong with these types of arrangements *per se*, as long as you're aware that they're NOT kindnesses:

They're mutually-beneficial business arrangements.

These types of business deals crop up all over the place in most of our social interactions. They're the unspoken rules you're following when you feel that you have to:

- Invite people back for a meal if they've invited you

- Ask people to come to your birthday bash or BBQ if they invited you

- Follow someone on Twitter, because now they're following you

- Buy a present for someone, if they got you one

- Babysit your neighbors' kids when they ask you, or do some other favor for them, because they've done you favors in the past

Again, there's nothing intrinsically wrong with these types of mutual business arrangements. They can even be really positive experiences, as long as both parties are completely clear from the start that they're participating in a deal with the terms: 'I will do this favor for you, on the understanding that you will reciprocate by doing X, Y and Z for me.'

The problems begin when people start passing off their business deals as an altruistic 'favor' or stand-alone kindness, but then attach a big, guilt-laden string to it.

When you get coerced into signing up for these sort of 'deals' without knowing what you're really getting into, it can cause you no end of heartache, stress, anxiety, guilt and other damaging negative emotions.

Why are 'strings' so bad?

This idea can be hard to grasp, so let's first restate the problem:

When you are entering into a mutually-beneficial arrangement that's completely aboveboard, i.e., both parties are up-front, honest and clear about what they are prepared to do, and what they expect to get in return, this shouldn't cause either party any emotional difficulties or issues whatsoever, and will probably also be really helpful and beneficial to them.

There are no strings in this scenario: it's a straight deal with clear terms, and both parties know exactly what they are agreeing to.

'Strings' occur when someone starts pretending that they are doing a kindness or favor for you completely altruistically, but then they attach an unspoken obligation or expectation to it that you should 'pay them back' in some way. They don't state this expectation up-front; they don't ask you if it's OK; and they don't give you any opportunity to discuss it, to see if you're actually comfortable with the 'payback' they want in return for the favor they're doing for you.

The main reason why this sort of manipulation can cause you tremendous anxiety is because it's effectively overriding your free choice. It's like being asked to sign a blank check: you have no idea what amount is going to get filled in, or when it's going to be presented back to you and you'll have to honor it, regardless of how many funds you actually have in your account.

Often what happens is that you'll be made to feel so guilty about the 'kindness' that was done for you in the past, that now you just *have* to comply with whatever request is being made of you, regardless of whether or not you actually *want* to do it.

Some very common examples of this could include:

- The in-laws who help pay for a holiday (or a car, or a new kitchen) for their children, on the unspoken condition that they then get to call the shots in their life.

- The elderly neighbor who goes out of her way to lend you things, but then starts using you as an unpaid taxi service, whenever she wants to go somewhere.

- The acquaintance who invites you for a meal, and then expects you to turn up for her big event to mark the 13th anniversary of her mother's death - whom you never actually met - because 'it's the least you could do.'

- The friend who shows up at your door with a plate of unexpected cookies, and then a little while later shows up again with her three kids and asks you to babysit for them for three hours, because she has a chore to do.

- The work colleague who covered for you when you came down with the flu, but who is now dumping a lot of their paperwork on your desk as 'payback.'

If you choose it, it's OK

Free choice is of paramount importance to us human beings. Free choice means that you:

1. Consciously understand 100% what's going on

2. Are genuinely choosing to participate in these types of arrangement

3. Fully understand all the 'strings' (i.e., expectations) involved

If these three conditions are met, then your 'favors' won't cause you any anxiety or difficulty and they could even be very beneficial for you.

But if you don't really understand what's happening, or you don't genuinely have free choice to make your own decisions about things, or you are made to feel guilty and obligated in some way; that's when you can get into all sorts of difficulties and your stress and anxiety levels can skyrocket.

> The third criteria for Appropriate Kindness: You have to really want to do the kindness and it shouldn't feel like an obligation or duty

Why appropriate kindness is a crucial foundation of your emotional health

Understanding what constitutes a genuine kindness is the key to maintaining your free choice, as well as your emotional health.

Emotions, particularly negative emotions, are not very popular these days. In today's modern world, you're increasingly being fed the line by pharmaceutical companies, psychiatrists and the medical establishment that there must be something fundamentally wrong with you if you feel bad, sad, down, overwhelmed, anxious, or angry.

(To give just one example, I recently read that the official psychiatric guidelines have been changed to state that if someone is still mourning the death of a loved one after TWO WEEKS, they should be treated as though they have clinical depression. By contrast, mourners are given a year to fully recover from a loved one dying, in the Jewish tradition.)

But negative emotions are part and parcel of the human experience, and as you learned previously, they normally contain some very important clues and signposts about what you need to change, work on, or address in your life, to truly fulfill your potential and be the person God created you to be.

When you react negatively to a person or to a situation it's nearly always because you feel hurt, upset, or threatened in some way.

Your negative emotion is just coming to show you that 'something' needs to change.

That 'something' could well be 100% internal, inside yourself, or it could be a prompt to make an external realignment or shift. Whatever the ultimate outcome, the key point to remember is that:

> *Your negative emotions contain messages and clues from God about what you need to work on, change or fix. But this amazing system of communication only works when you're actually aware of, and connected to, your authentic, deeper feelings.*

Kindness, or controlling?

When you're truly connected to your feelings, you can feel when something or someone is coming from a good place, or not. If you truly <u>feel</u> that a kindness is completely altruistic and string-free, then you'll also feel good and cared for when you receive it. But if you start to <u>feel</u> inexplicably weird, uncomfortable, or unhappy about the 'kindness' that's apparently being done for you, that's probably because, deep down, you have a gnawing sense that the other person is only doing kindnesses for you as a way of controlling you.

No one, not even the most generous, loving, compassionate kindhearted person, likes to feel like they are being controlled, manipulated or somehow taken advantage of. If this situation continues on for any length of time, it can cause some heavy-duty emotional and physical anxiety and stress.

Obligation or duty?

Some of the 'kindnesses' that you can be maneuvered into doing for others - which you fundamentally don't want to do - could include:

- The regular phone call you 'have' to make to a family member

- The visit you 'have' to make to someone

- The event or meeting you 'have' to attend

- The cake you 'have' to bake

- The favor you 'have' to do for someone, no matter how distasteful or inconvenient

- The chore or task that you're being forced to take on, even if you really don't want to do it.

When you tune into your inner dialogue, if you find the conversation is full of 'I HAVE to do this,' or 'I MUST do this,' or 'this is THE RIGHT THING TO DO' - these statements are very big indications that you're doing whatever it is out of a sense of obligation, and not because you really <u>want</u> to do it.

Again, occasional obligation is not a bad thing. But when your relationship with someone else is based almost exclusively on a sense of OBLIGATION, that's nearly always a clear sign that it's not a healthy relationship.

Want versus Should

When you really like or love someone, and they really like and / or love you, then you:

- WANT to spend time with them and vice versa

- WANT to talk to them

- WANT to do kindnesses for them

- WANT to help them out, because you actually ENJOY it.

> *It's: 'I WANT to do such and such,' not*
> *'I HAVE TO do such and such.'*

In an emotionally healthy relationship, you can be honest about the things that you actually don't want to do, without it causing a major breakdown in your relationship.

Which brings us neatly on to the next point:

> *You have to really WANT to do something,*
> *for it to count as a real kindness.*

Let's see how this plays out by zipping over to the local movie theater where, right now, some famous Hollywood star is acting out the role of a kind, compassionate husband and father.

In this scene, he's busy tucking his children lovingly into bed, with a kiss and a story. In that scene, he's painstakingly cooking supper for his wife, then he's off to visit the old-people's home, to play the accordion for the folks there to bring a bit of joy into their lives. What a saint this man apparently is! He's stuffed to the gills with good deeds...but it's all fake, it's all for show.

When the actor gets Upstairs and tries to claim some credit for his performance, they will waste no time in telling him that while it all looked so nice for the movie audience, spiritually, his good deeds counted for nothing. He was only acting nice; he wasn't feeling it in his heart.

And the same is true for all those 'kindnesses' and favors that you've been manipulated and coerced into doing, against your will.

Remember, free choice means that you can choose to say 'no.' If you feel that you can't say 'no' to someone even if you really want to - then you should explore how you may be being manipulated or scared into putting other people's interests and desires ahead of your own.

Watch out for the 'SHOULD'

So how can you know the difference between what you really want to be doing and what you're actually only doing grudgingly, because you can't seem to get out of it? That's a great question, but it can also be a very difficult one to truthfully answer.

The basic rule of thumb is this:

> *If you're using the word 'SHOULD,' that's a big clue that, really, you don't want to be doing whatever it is.*

Appropriate Kindness Also Applies to Doing Things for Yourself

Another frequently-overlooked area of appropriate kindnesses is the things that you can, and must, do for yourself. Many people have a funny idea that treating themselves nicely is somehow a selfish or lazy thing to do.

This can show up in many different areas – and you'll be able to identify more of your own areas of work as you continue along through the book – but treating yourself with appropriate kindness is probably the single best thing you could do to improve your happiness and health.

Let's give a few concrete examples of what I'm talking about. When you're treating yourself with appropriate kindness that means that you

DO:

- Judge yourself favorably, and give yourself the benefit of the doubt

- Recognize you have needs – even, a whole bunch of them

- Give yourself permission to buy the clothes you need, and to take the vacations you require, and to have the time and space you need to relax and nurture your soul, and to get a good night's sleep, etc.

Doing appropriate kindnesses for yourself also means that you

DON'T:

- Do things for other people that are going to harm you, in some way

- Don't beat yourself up

- Don't accuse yourself of being 'selfish,' or 'lazy,' when you have a long bath, sit down to read something, or book a much-needed massage

- Buy into the idea that doing kind things for yourself is somehow self-indulgent, or bad

The fourth criteria for Appropriate Kindness: It needs to come from a place of empathy and compassion

When you really want to do something, and it's coming from a place of wholehearted empathy and compassion, you normally feel happy, excited, good, and filled-up; even if what you want to do is very hard, and it's going to require a lot of time, energy and effort.

If you're genuinely choosing to do the kindness or favor, then AFTER you've done it, you'll feel on top of the world, your GodJuice will rev up, and you'll have tons of energy and enthusiasm.

By contrast, when you really don't want to be doing something, AFTER you've done it, you'll normally feel angry, resentful, depleted, tired, irritated, vengeful, frustrated, guilty and anxious when you think about it - even if it's the easiest thing in the world to do.

Instead of giving you strength, joy and a sense of profound satisfaction, the 'kindness' you were coerced into doing just sucked all the energy and GodJuice out of you, leaving you feeling miserable, stressed and drained.

When you don't make any attempts to look for the message these negative emotions are sending you and you leave them to fester, they can seriously impact your body and psyche, bringing you down and ultimately leading to any number of health issues. (In the second half of the book, you'll find a number of easy tools that will help you to start linking your specific negative emotions to specific health issues.)

Why you do things you don't really want to do

At one time or another, you probably got pulled into doing something that you really didn't want to do - or maybe, that you realistically weren't able to do - because you couldn't say no. It occasionally happens to all of us - but did you ever wonder why that is?

What switch got tripped in your unconscious mind to override your free choice and make you put other people's desires and feelings ahead of your own best interests?

You can sum the problem up succinctly in one sentence: *Children are notoriously easy to shame.* All an adult has to do is explode in anger at a child a few times for spilling the juice, or call them a moron for making a mistake, or criticize and belittle them when the child doesn't do exactly what the adult wants - and very quickly, kids end up programmed with subconscious 'override' buttons called: shame, guilt and fear.

When people press your 'toxic shame' button, or your 'fear' button, or your 'guilt' button to force you to do their will, they are effectively overriding your conscious free choice, and appealing straight to your subconscious fears. When you feel that you don't have free choice, or that you aren't being allowed to exercise it, your soul starts to choke and suffocate, because it can't fulfill its purpose in the world, namely CHOOSING to do good things.

Even if you're being forced to do a kindness or something that really does look, or even is genuinely good, your soul will still find the situation intolerable. In turn, this gives rise to all those negative emotions; like anger, vengeance, resentment, and maybe even a deep hatred of the person who is subconsciously forcing you to put their desires ahead of your own.

Let's see how this works in practice with a couple of common examples:

Examples of kindnesses that backfired

Eat your greens!

Larry was forced to eat his greens as a child, because his mother knew that broccoli and cabbage were healthy and good for him. Of course, Larry's mother was completely correct! But because Larry's free choice was repeatedly taken away from him in the area of eating his greens, the adult Larry still can't stand broccoli, even though, consciously, he's the first to admit that eating green, leafy vegetables would only benefit his health.

Self-service

Cara is a working mother with three young children. Cara's part of a community rota that makes meals for new mothers. Usually, Cara can manage the additional cooking, no sweat. But this week, she has a lot on her plate. Her own children have been ill and sleep-deprived for a few days in a row, she has a project deadline looming at work, and the missed sleep and extra pressure is making Cara feel pretty unwell herself. She's barely managing to cook for her own family, let alone anyone else.

But when her friend from the rota calls her to make a meal, Cara feels obliged to say 'yes.' For some reason, she feels that she just can't turn her friend down. That evening, the whole family tries to stay out of the kitchen as Cara is cooking. She's grouchy and irritable with everyone, and she's already angrily exploded a couple of times at her husband and kids.

We all know that these situations are just plain 'wrong.' But often that knowledge doesn't help us, and it only compounds our feeling of impotence and weakness that we couldn't just stand up for ourselves, making us feel even more confused, frustrated, tired, anxious and depleted.

Why you can't always 'Just say no'

When people lack compassion and empathy for others, they have no scruples about ruthlessly pressing any emotional button they can, in order to get the people in their life to do what they want. These unconscious buttons are at the root of all the manipulation and guilt tactics known to man, and it's the reason why you carry on saying 'yes' to some people when you dearly wish you could just say 'no.'

When someone has unhealthy emotional health habits, they often don't have the sense of accountability or compassion for others that would prevent them from pressing these buttons over and over again. The result is that many people get subconsciously forced into acting against their own best wishes, without understanding why it's making them feel so bad - or how they can stop it from happening in the future.

The good news...

The good news is that you can change this – you can disconnect these subconscious buttons, and regain your free choice again, by tackling the problem across all three levels of body, mind and soul.

At the soul level, you need to boost your GodJuice by talking to God about the issues you're facing. This may sound simplistic, but if you try it out for yourself you'll start to see some big shifts in your emotional state, and how you react to, and deal with, other people.

Appendix 2 at the back of this book contains a number of energy psychology exercises to help you defuse them at the emotional level.

And Appendix 1 at the back of the book has a wealth of energy medicine tips and techniques for how to deal with the body, or energetic, side of things.

HOW UNHEALTHY KINDNESSES CAN AFFECT YOUR HEALTH

When you feel like you have no choice, and that you have to go along with other people, regardless of what you actually want and prefer yourself, it can cause the following problems:

SPIRITUALLY: Every time you choose against yourself – i.e., you put other people's desires and wishes ahead of your own, deeper needs and inner truth - you disconnect yourself from your soul, i.e., the 'real you.' The more you disconnect from your soul, the harder it is to identify who the 'real you' is, or what you actually want.

Your soul is your interface with God, and it's how you recharge your GodJuice. When you become disconnected from your soul, your GodJuice can get very depleted and you can start to feel depressed, exhausted and despairing.

EMOTIONALLY: When other people are overriding your conscious free will by pressing your subconscious guilt, fear and toxic shame buttons, it can cause the following negative emotions (Please note: as so much of this is occurring at the subconscious level, these emotions are usually repressed, which can lead to blockages at the energetic level that can subsequently cause a number of physical issues.)

- Anger

- Anxiety

- Beating yourself up

- Depression

- Despair

- Emptiness

- Fear

- Feeling 'out of control'

- Guilt

- Hatred

- Indecision

- Loneliness

- Nervousness

- Obsession (e.g., you keep replaying conversations, etc., in your head)

- Panic

- Rage

- Resentment

- Self-hatred

- Shame

- Stress

- Worry

PHYSICALLY: As you'll learn throughout this book, repressed negative emotions are probably the number one reason why you get physically ill.

Each of your negative emotions is coming to teach you something. When you are disconnected from your true self, you also become disconnected from your true feelings. That means the 'message' goes undelivered, often causing a buildup of negative issues and toxic circumstances in your life.

In the Appendixes in the back of the book, you'll learn a number of easy to use, effective tools that can help you to unblock your emotions and meridians, at the physical level.

RECAP

- The Four Criteria of Appropriate Kindnesses are:

    1. It has to actually be experienced as a kindness by the recipient

    2. It should be 'string-free,' with no expectation of payback

    3. You have to really want to do it, i.e., it shouldn't feel like an obligation or duty

    4. It needs to come from a place of empathy and compassion

- Your negative emotions contain all sorts of messages and clues from God about how He wants you to act, and what He wants you to change. But this system only works when you're actually in touch with your true feelings.

- Whenever you phrase something to yourself as a '**SHOULD**' instead of as a '**WANT**,' that's a big, red flashing sign that you actually don't want to do it.

- Others can force us to 'choose against' our own best interests by pressing our subconscious emotional buttons, like guilt, fear, and shame.

Chapter 6

How Bad Influences Make Us Sick

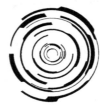

So far, you've learned how you can get sick when you get disconnected from God and your GodJuice dries up; and how unhealthy (or absent...) compassion, accountability and kindness can dissolve your spiritual energy, leading to all sorts of negative emotions and their associated health issues.

In this chapter, we're going to start widening out the net, to see what else may be making you ill, and what you can do about it. A little later on, you'll find some standard, 'no-brainer' stuff about environmental pollution, chemicals, junk food and electromagnetic smog; all topics that have been written about extensively by a number of other people. In the Resources section at the back of the book, you'll find a few recommendations for some further reading if you want to learn more.

But for most of this chapter, I want to concentrate on how the bad influences you're exposed to *socially* can damage your health as much, or even more than, the worst chemical pollutants or environmental hazards. Over the many years that I've been working with people to help them optimize their spiritual health, I've identified seven main categories of negative people, who can pull the rug out from under even the most emotionally-healthy person.

If you have only casual or infrequent interactions with these types of people, the damage they can do to you is pretty small. But if you're spending a lot of time with them, or if they're people who you're emotionally very connected to, their behavior and negative attitudes can take an enormous toll on your mental and physical health.

First, I'll tell you who they are and how they can affect you, and then I'll give you a bunch of practical advice on how you can minimize the health risks involved in hanging out with these folks.

The Seven Types of Negative People

1.   The Liar

How they can affect your health

Close your eyes, for a minute, and imagine that you've just caught your best friend / sibling / spouse / colleague lying to you about something emotionally significant. Maybe they 'borrowed' $50,000 out of your bank account without telling you... maybe they just stabbed you in the back and stole your idea for the 'deal of the century' right out from under your nose... maybe they just invited the whole neighborhood to their house for a big BBQ on the same day they knew you were planning to do it...

Now, what do you feel? Don't be shy! I won't tell anyone, I promise. This is just between the two of us.

What most of us would feel at this point is probably extreme anger and rage, mixed up with some jealousy, hatred, resentment, betrayal, disbelief, vengeance and enormous dislike. The liar is pretending to care about us, but they're not acting that way at all.

Do you know what a motherlode of pressure and physical stress all of these things put on your body? The racing heart, the hammering pulse, the tension headache, the neck pain, the tight chest, the back pain, the blurry eyesight, the raised blood pressure...

I could go on and on about how all of these things can lead directly to some serious physical illnesses (and when we get to the next chapter, I will).

But in the meantime, it should be clear that when you spend too much time with liars, particularly spiritually-unhealthy liars with minimal compassion, accountability and kindness, it can do you an awful lot of damage.

From a health perspective, chronic liars are so selfish, untrustworthy and unpredictable, that you'd have to be crazy to want to spend any time with them! Of course sometimes, you don't have any choice, especially if it's your boss or a close family member.

Does that mean that you're doomed to ill health? Not at all! You just have to recognize what you're dealing with, and take the appropriate steps to strengthen your own spiritual immune system, and energetic defenses. I'll tell you more about how to do this a little later on, when we get to the section on boundaries.

2.   The Competitor

How they can affect your health

Get ready...set...go!

How are you feeling as you power out of the blocks? Pumped up with adrenaline? Completely focused on getting ahead? No patience or time for any distractions (like your kids, for example...)?

There's a race to be won and you're not going to let anything get in your way.

How'd you feel if you made all that effort, and you still lost? How'd you feel if you lose every single time? Pretty bad, huh?

On the face of it, competition and competitors don't seem so bad. I mean, there is definitely a time and a place for that sort of striving and steely determination: just not all the time, and not every place. When you're constantly caught up in 'competing,' you're always just a nano-second away from tripping straight into the 'fight or flight' response, (more about this in the next chapter) which can put some serious stress on your body, your emotional health, and your relationships with others.

When you get caught up in 'competing,' you start boiling everything down to 'winning' or 'losing,' and the comparisons are endless: How much money am I earning, compared to so-and so? How much status do I have? Whose kids are doing better in school, mine or my sister's kids? Who's got the nicer garden, me or the neighbor? Who's eating the healthiest food? Who had the best vacation?

Hanging out with competitors can feel great when you're on the winning team. But when you're the one who feels like you're losing, you can get depressed and miserable very fast.

When you get caught up in competing, you get so focused on the outcome you rarely have any time or patience for the process. Trouble is, the 'process' can include a whole bunch of life-affirming, health-supporting things like playing with your kids, taking the time to nurture yourself, and talking to God.

3. The Classic Gossiper

How they can affect your health

You can sum it up like this: When you spend too much time with gossipers, it blows a huge hole in your self-esteem, your self-confidence and your integrity. (Did you *really* want the whole neighborhood to know that you just got unceremoniously dumped? Or fired?)

Healthy relationships and poisonous gossip very rarely go together. Healthy relationships are based on mutual independence and respect; seeing the good in others and encouraging others to believe in themselves and to develop their God-given talents and abilities to the max. Unhealthy relationships do exactly the opposite.

The more of these 'unhealthy' relationships you have, the less you usually actually like yourself, making you a whole lot more susceptible to unhelpful stuff like weight and food issues, 'self-soothing' bad habits and manipulative or 'control-freak' behavior.

I know that it can be so hard to stay away! There is often something almost addictive in being part of a gossip circle: think of the thrill we often get, despite ourselves, when we first hear the news of something shockingly bad. But the more gossip you're hearing, the less you'll find trust, consideration and care for others - and that's just not an encouraging, healthy vibe for you to be around.

4.   The Blamer

How they can affect your health

When people are walking around blaming and shaming all the time, there is NO healthy compassion going on.

Maybe it wouldn't be so bad if they were only blaming themselves, and leaving *you* alone. But blamers just aren't like that: they want to make sure that *you* also know that you're defective and simply not good enough.

When you keep getting blamed for a whole bunch of things that are actually not your responsibility (as discussed in the chapter on Sensible Accountability) - then you can really start to believe that *you* are the problem. If that continues to happen over any length of time, it's only natural that you'll start to dislike yourself for being so troublesome and problematic. I mean, if you weren't so darned stupid / incompetent / selfish / or thoughtless, everything would be just dandy!

And that is a classic recipe for a lot of emotional issues and physical problems, a little further down the road.

5.   The Mediator

How they can affect your health

I know what you're thinking: How can mediating between two warring parties be anything but good, kind, and healthy?

The truth is, sometimes it is. But that's not the sort of mediation I'm talking about here. I'm talking about the people who somehow manage to get themselves into the middle of your big crisis, or big dispute, or big problem, and then start turning it into a big theatrical 'Peace Now' event.

Instead of being about what you think, and about what you feel, your life starts to be run by an 'audience poll,' and that's really not good for your self-esteem or your clarity. That's because when there's so much politically correct 'peace and love' sloshing around, it can get really difficult to speak or act authentically, or to really be 'you.' You have to say what sounds good. You have to think acceptable thoughts.

The trouble is, repressed thoughts and feelings don't just disappear: they fester. The more we try to squash them down, instead of acknowledging them and dealing with them in a spiritually-healthy way, the greater the chances are that they'll show up as an energy block, emotional issue or even a physical problem, a little further on.

I know keeping the peace sounds very noble, but if you're not genuinely 'there' yet, it can be really, really bad for your health.

6.   The Worrier

How they can affect your health

Before you spent five minutes in the company of the worrier, you were feeling pretty upbeat, optimistic and happy about life. Now, you seem to have 'caught' their negative outlook, and you're starting to feel pretty stressed and worried.

- Maybe that bad cough your kid has is Ebola and you were really dumb not to go and get it checked out ASAP?

- Maybe that unopened letter from the bank is not just a routine statement, but is telling you they're foreclosing on your house?

- Maybe North Korea is going to try to set off a dirty-bomb in your neighborhood?

- Maybe the stock market really is going to crash through the floor today, and wipe out your retirement fund?

On and on it goes. Instead of smiling and enjoying the roses, now you're consumed with anxiety and stress. Ten seconds later, your neck starts hurting, you get a migraine spike, your back starts twinging, or you start to feel really weak on one side of your body...

Nothing can make your energy and good health nose-dive faster than fear and negativity - and worriers excel at combining both of these things into an emotionally-lethal cocktail. When you believe that everything comes down to random statistics, freak weather, terrorists and mutant bacteria - you worry. A lot.

When you worry about too many things too much of the time, you create an emotional environment where nasty things like fatigue, stress, pain, deep pessimism and futility can take hold and flourish.

But when you start trying to believe that God is running the world, you stop worrying so much and you start to feel a whole lot better.

7.   The Mocker

How they can affect your health

When you're sincerely trying to be a better person, or to get closer to God, or to improve your circumstances, (you bought this book, I'm talking about you here!) few things can torpedo your ability to aspire, improve and to change faster or more effectively than being mocked.

It only takes one particularly sharp comment, or one run-in with a cruel, shameless 'smart mouth' to wipe out a whole bunch of your healthy energy and leave you feeling half-dead. That's why the best advice for mockers is to stay as far away from them as you can. Period.

Of course, you're not always in control of the people in your environment and even if you're doing your best to stay away from callous cynics, you may still have to deal with them in your workplace, or your place of worship, or at the bank.

The good news is there's still a bunch of things you can do to protect yourself from all their unhealthy vibes, as we're about to find out.

Minimizing the fallout from negative people

In keeping with what we've already identified as being the three main reasons why you get sick, the coping strategy for dealing with negative people is split into three main parts:

1.   **The 'Talking to God' solution**

2.   **The 'Maintaining Good Emotional Health' solution**, and lastly, what I'll call

3.   **The 'Mobilizing the Good Energy Defense' solution**, that's connected to a lot of the information you'll find a little later on, in the second part of the book, where we'll discuss energy meridians.

A small word of warning: some of the following ideas may sound distinctly weird, but please don't let that put you off from trying them. None of these things can do you any harm, and they really could help a lot to shore up your spiritual and physical strength and keep your good energy humming.

1) THE 'TALKING TO GOD' SOLUTION

This one's really pretty simple to do, and probably the easiest of the lot: ask God to keep all the worst crazies away from you, as much as possible. Remember, miracles can and do happen!

If they're still managing to slip under your radar, you can also ask God to help you implement the next few suggestions, to help you to cope with them and minimize any damage they might be doing to you.

2) THE 'MAINTAINING GOOD EMOTIONAL HEALTH' SOLUTION

The key thing all of the following ideas have in common is that they help you to set up, and maintain, healthy boundaries. Putting up and policing firm boundaries doesn't happen overnight. It's a process, and it will take some time to start doing these things consistently and routinely, especially if you've made it your life's work to get stepped on, bossed around and generally taken advantage of up until now.

So celebrate every small step you make in creating a healthier emotional environment for yourself. If you get stuck at any point, simply take it back to God, and let Him help you deal with it. Just remember: God's got your back...

So without any further ado, here are my tips for how to maintain good emotional health:

I. Maintain firm boundaries

II. Don't blame yourself

III. Hang out with positive people

I - Put Firm Boundaries in Place, Using the Following Three Rules

Rule 1: Accept that not everyone is nice

You would be amazed at how many people get stuck on this basic idea, even though they may have been hurt, misled, mistreated or otherwise abused countless number of times. No one likes to look at the bad. No one likes to think that they may be living in a world full of not-so-nice individuals. It makes us feel kind of...icky.

But if you don't accept the reality that not everyone you know, like, or work with has a conscience and that not everyone out there acts, thinks or believes in the same way you do, your health and well-being could really suffer, as a result.

When people are repeatedly making you feel 'bad,' 'selfish,' 'in the wrong,' or that you are responsible for somehow fixing their problems, their issues or their life, it's a big, flashing red sign that something is severely wrong here, spiritually.

If you're picking up that vibe, don't argue with it! Ignoring the hints that your soul is repeatedly trying to give you can lead to some big feelings of anxiety, fear and stress, and eventually, it can also lead to illness. Hard as it may be, accept that some people aren't very nice and that you could be dealing with someone who has some very big problems.

Once you do that, you'll already start to feel a whole lot better: more protected, safer, and more empowered and in control of your interactions, along with feeling much more resilient to getting hurt or being manipulated. The crazies will feel that something's changed in their interaction with you, and they'll start to leave you alone and be much less in your face (and if you're *really* lucky, they'll retire and move to the other side of the country).

Rule 2: Learn to trust your gut instincts

Probably the single biggest thing that will stop you from implementing Rule 1 (once you come out of denial about the existence of bad people in the world) is that you don't always know who is actually good for you, and who isn't. Part of the reason it can be so confusing is because some bad people go to great lengths to curry favor and appear kind and trustworthy. If you're feeling confused and unsure of what's really going on with your relationships, take a time-out and listen to your feelings. How is your gut reacting to this person? Is your relationship more about WANT, or is it more about SHOULD?

Do you WANT to spend time with them, talk to them, do favors for them, or do you feel somehow obliged to them, like you SHOULD be around them, or helping them out? Are you scared of their reaction if you say 'no' to their requests, or go against them in some way? Are you worried they might start bad-mouthing you? Do they regularly bad-mouth other people? Do you feel intimidated or threatened by them, like you wouldn't put it past them to overreact and try to do something nasty to 'punish you' for not toeing their line? Do they make you feel genuinely good about yourself, or bad? Are they highly critical of the people around them? Is it always about 'them'?

Listen to the message your intuition is trying to tell you, particularly if you get a sense that 'something' is a bit off, or doesn't quite add up about the person.

Our gut feelings about people are usually very accurate, but our social conditioning presses the override button, because we don't want to be seen as rude or unaccommodating. But it's a million times better to walk away from bad, than to get mugged by it.

Rule 3: Walk away

I know that a lot of crazies can be funny, charming and entertaining, at least occasionally. But we have to weigh all the 'excitement' and color they can inject into our lives against all the stress that comes along with people who routinely lie, compete, gossip, blame, 'peace-seek,' worry or ridicule others. Think of these crazies as being like emotional MSG: sure, they spice up whatever action, environment or relationship they find themselves in, but they can still give you brain damage...

Feel free to 'treat' yourself, occasionally, to whatever flavor of mental madness most takes your fancy, but if you ever suspect it might be harming your health, do whatever you need to do to protect yourself.

Example: Eli the Bad Friend

From the moment she met him, Rachel couldn't stand her husband Michael's friend Eli. Eli was a few years older than her husband, and was full of colorful stories about all the daring missions he'd undertaken for the army and all the crazy things he'd been involved with.

Although Eli could talk the hind legs off a donkey, he seemed very disinterested in what Michael was up to, and hardly ever had a word for Rachel, beyond asking her to make him a cup of coffee whenever he came around.

Eli's stories always made him sound like a big-hearted angel of mercy, who was constantly looking for people to help and good causes to support. But in practice, every time he popped around (usually without any prior notice), his egotistical behavior and palpable arrogance left a nasty taste in Rachel's mouth. The final straw came when Rachel 'caught' Michael handing over a few hundred dollars, when she unexpectedly came out to hand him the phone, as he was saying good-bye to his friend on the doorstep.

As soon as Eli drove off, Rachel asked Michael to tell her what was going on. It turned out that Eli had been recently fired (again), and was struggling to make ends meet. Michael had been helping him out with a few hundred dollars for the last few weeks.

Rachel hit the roof: why hadn't Michael mentioned it to her? Michael started to feel very confused, and explained that he knew that Rachel didn't like Eli, so when Eli suggested they keep it 'just between the two of us,' he was more than happy to agree.

Rachel looked her husband squarely in the eyes: "Michael, can't you see how all of this just doesn't add up? If he's so great, and wonderful, and involved in all these good deeds, like he keeps telling you, why can't he hold down a job? Why's he been divorced twice? Why do I never hear him talking about his kids, or asking you about what's going on in your life? Can't you see that he's just taking you for a ride?"

Michael tried to explain that it wasn't like that, and that Eli had been through a lot of things that Rachel didn't know about. He'd had a lot of bad luck. People didn't understand him. But the explanations fell a bit flat, even to his own ears. Later, in a quiet moment, a very confused Michael tried to sort through all of his conflicting thoughts and feelings. What was *really* going on with Eli?

II - Don't Blame Yourself for the Problem

It's not your responsibility (or fault) if others are unhappy and negative. You don't have to 'fix' other people - and even if you want to, you can't! Each of us is responsible for our own outlook and happiness, so don't let a negative person make *their* problem, *your* problem. If they're unhappy, keep your distance until they calm down again, and try not to take it personally when they start griping, blaming, raging, controlling and manipulating.

III - Hang Out With People Who Exude Positivity

You know how we said that negativity is infectious? Well, so is happiness! I promise you that happy people who are spiritually healthy do still exist, and can still be found. (Here's one idea: hang out in your local bookstore and see who else is drawn to this book...)

That old adage is true: birds of a feather flock together. As your own spiritual health starts to improve, you'll start to attract tons of like-minded caring, compassionate, kind and responsible people into your life. Your spirit will soar, your social life will rock, and your health will be the best it's ever been, at every level.

3) THE 'MOBILIZING THE GOOD ENERGY DEFENSE' SOLUTION

OK, you've talked to God about getting the energy-sucking jerk in the next cubicle relocated to the office in Australia and you've done your best to put up good boundaries and to start hanging out with nicer people. But at least every now and then, you'll still find yourself spending time with a negative type. When that occurs, try the following tips to minimize their energetic fallout:

1) Carry Your Invisible Umbrella

If you know in advance you're dealing with a difficult person who sucks you dry and exhausts you, keep them out of your personal space as much as possible. Put up your 'invisible umbrella' to keep people at arm's length; if they're trying to hug you, stand too close to you, pat your arm, etc., then gently move away, so they're no closer to you than they would be if you were holding an umbrella. Don't be scared to police your invisible boundary forcefully, if you have to. They'll get the message sooner or later.

2) Take a Shower

Before and / or after you have to deal with someone you know is 'difficult,' take a shower. Energetically, nothing washes away residual negativity faster than a bit of hot water and soap.

3) Place Them on Your Right-Hand Side

Energetically-speaking, you are wired to absorb far more of the stuff coming in from your external environment on the left side of your body. That means that you're much more vulnerable to negative factors coming in from that direction. When 'the problem' is on your right (whoever or whatever that may be), you'll find it so much easier to bat away anything that isn't useful or helpful.

4) Cross Your Arms

Many people already do this automatically, whenever they're around some-one who's a bit 'too much' for them, for whatever reason. There's a good reason for why they do this: it works! Energetically-speaking, it helps you to feel more secure and self-contained, and less open to other people's antics and bad energy.

(As a side note, having the urge to cross your arms when you're near someone doesn't automatically mean that they're bad for you; you could genuinely love them to bits and really enjoy their company, but still sometimes find them a little bit overwhelming.)

5) Take a Bath in Baking Soda

I *know* this sounds mega-weird, but it really does help a person feel more grounded, 'together' and cleaned-up from all the emotional 'ick.'

6) Try the Following Energy Medicine Exercises

While this book is much more about optimizing your spiritual health than about Energy Medicine, I think it's still appropriate to bring in a couple of great energy exercises here. These exercises can help you to strengthen your:

- GodJuice, by connecting you directly back to God

- Spiritual and emotional energy, by helping you to create good boundaries

- Physical energy and fitness, by helping you to process all the 'environmental pollution' your body has to deal with, every single day.

The 'God Is Everywhere' Energy Exercise

- Rub your hands together, and shake them off.

- Rub them together again, and then put the palms facing either side of your ears.

- Bring your elbows together in front your face, and then cross your arms over each other, so that your hands sweep past your face (palms facing your face), then continue to sweep your arms out to the side.

- Cross your arms over in front of you again, and again sweep them out to the side. Do these crisscross movements in front of you all the way down your body and legs, until you get to the floor.

- Have in mind that God is protecting you, and keeping you cocooned-off in His kindness and light.

- When you reach the floor, put your two arms together, kind of like an elephant's trunk, and make sweeping figure 8 movements around your body, as you come back up from your legs to your head.

- Take the figure 8 movements up past your head, then put your two arms together, backs of hands touching, above your head, and then bring them gently down to the sides of your body.

- Imagine as you do this, that you are literally in a cocoon of Divine protection.

The 'Give It Back to God' Energy Exercise

- Rub your hands together and shake them off.

- Bring your hands together in front of your chest, palms touching.

- Zoom one hand up, palm up to God, and zoom one hand down, palm down, as though you're pressing against the ground (you're not really touching the ground, though, you stay standing up straight). Stretch.

- Now, switch sides - zoom the 'up' hand to the 'down' position, and vice versa.

- While you're doing this, have in mind that you are giving whatever you need to back to God, to take care of, while retaining whatever experience, learning or 'good' you need to keep hold of.

- Do this twice more on both sides.

- Then bend over with your arms down in front of you and take two deep breaths.

- Now, slowly stand up, rolling your arms up your body as you do so. (Imagine you're rolling a beach ball up your body).

- Take your arms above your head, and bring them down to your sides.

- Imagine, as you do this, that God is covering you in a protective mantle of Divine light.

Other Bad Influences That Can Make You Sick

The focus of this book is primarily on how to maintain and optimize your spiritual and emotional health, so that you don't end up physically ill. That said, your physical actions and lifestyle choices can also make you physically ill (like, duh!) and, perhaps more surprisingly, they can also make you emotionally and spiritually sick, too.

The general rule of thumb is:

> *The more you minimize the 'nasties' coming in from outside, the stronger, happier and healthier you'll be - but don't get all fanatical about it.*

One of the main reasons I wanted to write this book is because I've seen so many people get swept up in the 'rightness' of their healthy lifestyle choices that they lose all perspective on what's *really* going to keep them feeling great.

Sure, it's wonderful to eat organic food and filter all your water. But please don't start beating yourself up for that occasional bar of chocolate or big steak dinner, because when you get down on yourself like that, you get flooded with negative emotions, you cut yourself off from God and you end up doing far more damage to yourself, health-wise, than that poor piece of cow could ever have done in a million years.

So to sum it up: All of the following are all definitely bad for you and should be minimized as much as possible. But if forgoing your Starbucks is going to get you all sad and depressed – then go ahead and buy the double chocolate macchiato and enjoy it! Bear in mind that the stronger the Divine energy, aka GodJuice, you have flowing through your body, and the better your emotional health is, the more you can handle the other elements and unhealthy substances that could otherwise really throw your health for a loop.

Got it? Great! Let's move on, then. Things to minimize and avoid as much as possible include:

Environmental Pollution

It's best not to live right next to the busiest highway in the country, on top of a nuclear reactor, or in a place where your neighbors regularly enjoy setting fire to the garbage.

Junk Food

Like we said, eating a little bit of something technically 'bad' for you is not the end of the world, as long as you enjoy it tremendously and don't start beating yourself up because of it. But you are what you eat - once you're done digesting it all, it literally turns into your body, your bones, and your brain - and high-quality input will produce much higher-quality health.

Food additives, E-numbers, food colorings and the dreaded MSG - these things can all play havoc with your health, particularly if you're disconnected from God and full of negative emotions. You want the food you eat to give you energy, not to drain all of the energy out of you, give you acne and leave you with an extra 30 pounds to lug around.

Electromagnetic Smog

I know you really don't want to hear this, but i-Phones, internet, laptops, tablets, microwaves - they all give off a lot of electromagnetic smog that the body then has to try to deal with and process.

The same rules of thumb apply: If the other areas of your life are generally healthy, and your energy levels are high to begin with, you'll probably be able to manage the additional electromagnetic processing OK. If that's not the case, every additional processing 'chore' is putting more strain on your already overburdened system and, if you don't get your system more in balance, then sooner or later you'll crack and could wind up ill.

You don't have to throw out all your favorite electronic gadgets, (although there are some people who'd disagree with me...) but it's wise to limit the amount of electromagnetic smog you're exposing yourself to, in any way you can.

In a number of scientific experiments, the sort of electromagnetic doses that every single one of us is exposed to *every single day,* just by going to work and being in our home environments, was shown to cause a number of physiological changes in the way the body operates; affecting everything from hormone production, to eyesight, to the reproduction and division of cells.

Many of these changes are distinctly unhealthy, and are being linked to some very nasty diseases. (Let's put it like this: If there wasn't such a huge vested financial interest behind our hi-tech lifestyle, most countries would have banned computers, TVs, radio stations and microwaves a long time ago..).

You'll only help your health by doing whatever you can do to 'disconnect' – within reason. Then, don't sweat it, because God is running the world.

Chemicals

Today, there's something like 17,000 different chemicals just in the food you eat. But that's not the only place they're cropping up: they're in your shampoo, your detergent, your makeup, your body care products, your clothing, your furnishings, your cleaning products...you get the idea.

Once again, I'm not advocating an all-or-nothing approach, but the fewer chemicals your body has to deal with, the more energy you'll have available for fun things like going to the beach.

It's getting easier and easier to find more natural alternatives to many of the chemical-laden products we eat, use and buy. If you can easily find a healthier alternative, and it won't bother you to make the change, go for it! The trick to getting this to really work for you, without feeling like you're missing out on the things you love, is to find out what level of toxins, chemicals or environmental 'stress' your body can actually handle, before it makes you sick.

Once you have a rough idea of what your tolerance level actually is, and what all this stuff may actually be doing to your health, then you can sit down and prioritize which additives, toxins and stresses you won't miss, and which ones you really can't do without.

Personally, I'm happy to use a simpler shampoo and a more environmentally-friendly detergent for my laundry, but I draw the line at chemical-free deodorants that don't work and leave me smelling like someone's old shoe.

Remember: God's got your back. That means that you don't have to do all this stuff perfectly. When God's behind you, you can continue with some of your ill-health inducing bad habits and know it's still going to be fine.

Most days I have my green smoothie for breakfast, but some days, I eat a whole chocolate bar instead. When that happens, I enjoy the change, I don't beat myself up about it, and I remind myself that God's running the world, and looking after my health. And if I skip the parsley-avocado-date shake every once in a while because the Hershey bar is calling to me, it's OK.

The last thing to say about chemicals is that conventional drugs and medications are chock-full of them. Even the lowly aspirin is actually a super-potent, powerful chemical in a very concentrated form. Again, if the drug is saving your life, there's nothing to discuss. If it isn't, consider a healthier, less risky alternative and take that additional toxic load off your system, and out of your body.

We each need all the energy we can get our hands on in order to stay fit and healthy. Once you've done your best to remove, stop or reduce whatever's blocking your energy at the spiritual and emotional level, that often leads to some dramatic and permanent improvements in many of your physical issues, without you having to make a lot of changes in other areas of your life.

RECAP

The following Seven Types of Negative People can really affect your health:

1. The Liar

2. The Competitor

3. The Classic Gossiper

4. The Blamer

5. The Mediator

6. The Worrier

7. The Mocker

The 3 Rules of Putting Firm Boundaries in Place Are:

1. Accept that not everyone is nice.

2. Learn to trust your gut instincts.

3. Walk away.

Other environmental influences that you should also try to minimize include:

- Junk Food

- Environmental Pollution

- Electromagnetic Smog

- Chemicals

The general rule of thumb is:

> *The more you minimize the 'nasties' coming in from outside, the stronger, happier and healthier you'll be - but don't get all fanatical about it.*

Chapter 7

Meridians - The Energy of Emotions

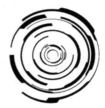

What are 'Energy Meridians?'

Energy meridians were first mapped in the human body around 3,500 years ago by Chinese physicians, who understood that some sort of subtle energy (what we would call the soul) was animating the body.

When this energy was flowing around the body correctly, the person stayed healthy. When the energy was stuck, stagnant, weak or blocked in some way, the person got sick.

These early practitioners of Chinese medicine mapped the energy flow around the body and identified 14 main energy 'pathways,' which they called meridians. Each meridian was named for the main organ, or physical system, it governed or regulated in the body.

They then developed the systems of acupuncture (using small needles inserted into particular points along each meridian) and acupressure (using light pressure from the fingers on certain points along each meridian) to help energy flow better, and to help release the energetic 'blocks' in the body. From the beginning, Chinese medicine recognized that the energetic blocks in the body were usually caused by the person's emotions.

Many, many books have been written about Chinese medicine, 5 Element Theory, acupuncture, acupressure and the energy meridians. In the Resources section at the back of this book, you'll find some recommendations for further reading.

The energy of emotions

What we're going to concentrate on in this chapter, is how to identify the emotional energy that's behind each meridian. The 'Talking to God' approach is to look for the real root of your health problem, according to the following, three-pronged approach that we've been setting out throughout this book:

1) Check Your Connection To God. If it's lacking, or very weak, this is the first place that needs work. A poor, weak or absent connection to God equates to you having no or very little Divine energy, or GodJuice, flowing through your body.

2) Check Your Emotional Health-o-Meter against the three foundations of good emotional health, as described in chapters 4-6. The three foundations of emotional health are:

1. Healthy compassion

2. Sensible accountability

3. Appropriate kindness

If all three of these areas are balanced and healthy, your emotional energy should be strong and flowing well around all areas of your body.

3) Check What Particular Spiritual or Emotional Issue Might Be Causing A Physical Health Problem. In this third stage of the process, you need to do some detective work to try to find out what specific issue or problem God is trying to resolve, or bring to your attention, via a specific illness or health issue. And in many cases, your emotions will hold the key to discovering the answer.

I know that idea can sound a bit surprising, or even a bit weird. I mean, you're probably used to a medical reality where the first thing you do when you get sick is get a bunch of tests done to see what's going on with your biology, like your blood, your glucose, your cholesterol levels, etc.

But in the talking to God approach, we're not so interested in what's gone wrong, we want to know why it's gone wrong in the first place. What emotion is being repressed or reacted to, when you reach for the chips? And that's where the meridians can really help you.

For example, you don't need to be a rocket scientist to know that eating bad food makes a person ill. But now, you're interested in finding out *why* you're being drawn to the bad food in the first place. What emotion are you repressing, or reacting to unconsciously, when you're reaching for the chips? And that's where the meridians can help really you.

Ask someone to help you, or Do-It-Yourself

In clinical settings that offer meridian-based therapies like applied kinesiology, acupuncture and acupressure, there are a number of relatively easy, safe and non-invasive diagnostic exercises you can do to find out which of your energy meridians are 'out' in some way. Then, it's usually pretty easy to work back from there, to identify the emotional blocks that may be behind the physical problems.

But one of the main reasons I wrote this book is because I wanted to help you, the reader, to take your health back 'in-house,' and to give you the tools you need to help you work out the answers to why you're really getting sick, by yourself.

This chapter contains a lot information and ideas, (which can be a bit scary-looking and intimidating at first) but once you start to read it, you'll find that it's organized very simply, and that it's actually pretty user-friendly.

To avoid throwing too much stuff at you at once, I've put the technical information on how to use simple acupressure techniques to balance and unblock your meridians into Appendix 1, at the back of the book.

I've also included some very simple self-diagnostic tools in the next chapter, which will hopefully make it even easier for you to see where your energy might be getting blocked. I've also included my top tips, tools and techniques for what you can do to get it flowing again.

If you're feeling a bit overwhelmed by all the new concepts and information, then by all means consider going to a reputable, God-fearing practitioner who works with meridians, to get the ball rolling. But even if you decide to outsource some of this work to someone else, remember that YOU are still the most powerful, knowledgeable and effective person involved in your own healthcare. Nobody knows you like you do, and no one is more interested and committed to maintaining your health.

How to activate your internal 'Energy Detective'

The key requirement for every successful 'Energy Detective' is an inquiring mind. Practically speaking, that means that you'll need to:

- Be willing to ask yourself some hard questions

- Follow every lead that comes up, even if initially it doesn't look very promising or likely

- Be prepared to brainstorm with your nearest-and-dearest (and to actually listen to what they're telling you...) if you find yourself getting stuck down a blind alley and you can't seem to find the exit.

If all else fails, radio your Superior for help (i.e., go and talk to God about it all) and He'll send you the next clue you need to work out what's really going on with your health, and why. But keep your eyes open, as God's hints are not always so obvious, or easy to spot. They can literally come from any direction, or via any interaction you have, even apparently random chance meetings and throw-away comments.

If this is starting to sound too much like hard work, take heart - working out what's really making you sick is like winning at Cluedo - but about five million times better. You'll feel so gratified, energized and empowered when you've finally managed to successfully piece together all the parts of your health puzzle.

There is simply no greater feeling than getting healthier, getting more self-empowered and self-aware, and getting closer to God.

Right, detective, are you ready for your first case? Great. Let's begin.

Where is the block?

The first mystery you need to solve is:

> *Where is the specific problem, or block, occurring, and what meridians do you need to work with to get it freed up?*

If you already know that you have a physical problem, or a physical weakness in a particular area of your body, then it's pretty easy to work this part of the equation out. In the Quick Reference Table on page 185 you'll find a bunch of the most common physical issues that can occur when the energy is weak, unbalanced or blocked in a particular meridian.

Simply check through the Table to find your illness, organ or specific issue, then go straight to the relevant meridian, to see what emotional issues or 'lost' feelings may be hiding underneath.

The Table doesn't include an exhaustive list of illnesses, and it doesn't need to, because your intuition and talking to God also play a big part in working out what's really making you ill, and finding the true underlying cause.

If your particular illness isn't listed, or you don't have any specific physical illnesses or issues, begin by reading through the following descriptions of the different emotional states associated with each specific meridian. As you go through, I'm sure at least one or two will jump out at you as being possible candidates. Start there, work with those meridians, and see if things start to unblock, shift and clear.

If you're still stuck, stumped or blocked, try the diagnostic quizzes in the next chapter to see if they shed some more light on your particular situation or illness. If they don't, go back to God and ask for more clues. If you're sincerely searching for the answers, sooner or later, you will find them.

There's always an exception to the rule

The information presented in this chapter is just a jumping-off point. If something doesn't sound right, or doesn't work for you, that's OK! We are all unique creations, and there will be exceptions to the rule. Also, as I keep on stressing, the real healing comes when you take your issues or problems back to God and ask Him to help you resolve them.

So the information presented below should be used as an accurate but general guide to finding out what emotional and spiritual 'blocks' might be behind your physical problems, but the last word, as always, rests with you. You are responsible for your health, and you can know far more about yourself, and your issues, and your blocks, than any outside expert, especially if you're regularly checking in with God to see what's really going on.

With all those caveats out of the way, let's start by naming the 14 main energy meridians in the body, and the main primary emotions they're associated with.[1]

The 14 meridians - An Emotional Overview

CENTRAL MERIDIAN - Emotional energy when unbalanced: feeling vulnerable or 'lacking.' Emotional energy when balanced: Feeling grounded, confident and secure.

GOVERNING MERIDIAN - Emotional energy when unbalanced: unable to move forward, 'no backbone.' Emotional energy when balanced: 'can do-ability,' having the courage to move on, overcome problems and try new things.

STOMACH MERIDIAN - Emotional energy when unbalanced: anxiety, pessimism and extreme worry about day-to-day problems and needs. Emotional energy when balanced: trusting that everything will turn out OK, calm and serene and a strong belief in God's goodness.

SPLEEN MERIDIAN - Emotional energy when unbalanced: either too much compassion for others and too little for the self, or too little compassion for others and too much for the self, or too little compassion for anyone and unable to accept and internalize others' ideas, feelings, or needs. Emotional energy when balanced: compassionate and caring, fair and generous with others but not at the expense of the self, able to assimilate and respond to 'outside' information.

HEART MERIDIAN - Emotional energy when unbalanced: heartache or a broken heart. Emotional energy when balanced: love, seeing the good in the self and others.

SMALL INTESTINE MERIDIAN - Emotional energy when unbalanced: pulled all over the place, confusion, unable to make decisions. Emotional energy when balanced: can act decisively and know what you want.

---

1   Much of the information in this chapter was inspired by the work of Donna Eden and David Feinstein.

BLADDER MERIDIAN - Emotional energy when unbalanced: Fearful of the outside world, despairing, pessimistic. Emotional energy when balanced: Strong belief in God's goodness, optimistic, trusting, courageous.

KIDNEY MERIDIAN - Emotional energy when unbalanced: loneliness, ashamed of the self, traumatized, 'frozen,' existential angst. Emotional energy when balanced: deep acceptance of the self, strong, healthy connections to others, strong connection to God.

CIRCULATION-SEX MERIDIAN - Emotional energy when unbalanced: frustrated by 'over choice,' too many demands, ignores their own deepest emotional needs, commitment-phobic. Emotional energy when balanced: has healthy priorities, recognizes and responds to their emotional needs, committed.

TRIPLE WARMER MERIDIAN - Emotional energy when unbalanced: heavy-duty stress, the 'fight / flight / freeze' response, aka 'I'm taking control, here, and looking after Number 1.' The Triple Warmer Meridian's main emotions are primal fear and self-preservation. Nothing can kill our joy and our connection to God as fast and as effectively as a rampaging Triple Warmer. Emotional energy when balanced: feeling safe and secure, humbly trusting God's goodness.

GALLBLADDER MERIDIAN - Emotional energy when unbalanced: anger at others, very judgmental and critical, unforgiving, demanding. Emotional energy when balanced: kind, merciful, tolerant and forgiving, with healthy assertiveness.

LIVER MERIDIAN - Emotional energy when unbalanced: 'beating ourselves up,' hyper-critical of the self, guilt feelings. Emotional energy when balanced: positive feelings about the self, self-forgiveness and acceptance, able to nurture and care for the self.

LUNG MERIDIAN - Emotional energy when unbalanced: profound sadness and grief, yearning, unwillingness to get emotionally involved with others, aloof. Emotional energy when balanced: belief in God's goodness, renewal, excitement, an ability to let go and move on, ability to connect to others at the deepest levels.

LARGE INTESTINE MERIDIAN - Emotional energy when unbalanced: control-freak, a need to be in control, even when it's damaging the self and others. Emotional energy when balanced: surrenders control, can let go of outmoded, unneeded, or toxic things.

The 14 Meridians In Detail

Note: Unlike the other 12 meridians, the Central and Governing Meridians relate to the overall energy and general well-being of a person, as opposed to a specific organ and / or function in the body, or specific emotion.

Central Meridian- *Emotional energy when unbalanced: feeling vulnerable or 'lacking.' Emotional energy when balanced: feeling grounded, confident and secure.*

Central

Thanks to its close connection with the brain and the nervous system, Central Meridian is generally involved with all matters of the mind. Whenever you're hoping for something to happen, or you're trying to believe in something or someone (including yourself), Central Meridian will be activated. The Central Meridian is the most suitable meridian for self-suggestion and hypnosis.

When the GodJuice in the Central Meridian is flowing well, you:

■ Can easily let go of ideas, emotions, beliefs, truths and even physical objects and things that may have served you well in the past, but which have now outlived their usefulness.

■ Can take in and accept new ideas, beliefs and truths, and maintain a flexible outlook and attitude to life.

■ Don't get stuck in the past; you 'flow with the tide' and easily tailor and adapt your outlook to new circumstances and different demands.

■ Feel confident and secure in your ability to handle whatever life has in store for you, which means that you enjoy the ebb and flow in your life.

■ Continue to evolve and grow as circumstances (and God) dictate.

When the GodJuice in Central Meridian is blocked or unbalanced, you can experience the following issues:

■ Spend too much time 'over-thinking' and over-analyzing

- Find it hard to 'get out of your head'

- Live life in theory, instead of in practice

- Brain fatigue

- Learning difficulties

- Feelings of anxiety and stress

- Can feel very vulnerable, especially in social settings

- Scared of, or paralyzed by the idea of change

> *Governing Meridian - Emotional energy when unbalanced: unable to move forward, 'no backbone.' Emotional energy when balanced: 'can-do ability,' having the courage to move on, overcome problems and try new things.*

Governing

Like the Central Meridian, Governing Meridian is also directly plugged in to your central nervous system and deals with 'global' effects in the body and soul.

The Governing Meridian runs along the backbone, and is related to your general sense of confidence and courage.

When the GodJuice in the Governing Meridian is flowing well, you:

- Can move forward in life, even when facing some big obstacles.

- Have the courage and strength you need to fully engage with, and participate in your family life, community, and the outside world.

- Have good posture; you will literally stand up straight, and hold your head high.

When the GodJuice in Governing Meridian is blocked or unbalanced, you can experience the following issues:

- Slumped or poor posture

- Issues with the pineal gland (particularly issues pertaining to light and darkness)

- Feeling overburdened

- Feeling stuck, or feeling like you're going in reverse

- Feeling spineless or clueless, or lacking in courage to change something or move forward

> *Stomach Meridian* - *Emotional energy when unbalanced: anxiety, pessimism and extreme worry about day-to-day problems and needs. Emotional energy when balanced: trusting that everything will turn out OK, calm and serene with a strong belief in God's goodness.*

Stomach

All the meridians are connected to, are affected by and also influence our emotions. Stomach Meridian is the most 'emotional' meridian of them all. Emotional issues often hit the Stomach Meridian the fastest, and the hardest.

When the GodJuice in the Stomach Meridian is flowing well, you:

- Have confidence that things will work out and you're not afraid to break out of the status quo and try new things.

- Have a profound sense that God is in the picture, and that whatever happens, you can trust Him to come through for you to ensure that you'll always have what you need to perform your mission in life. This gives you the confidence to be out in the world, and to be open to new ideas, options and things.

- Feel full, satisfied, content, calm, relaxed and happy.

- Trust that God is looking after you and that He's going to meet all of your needs, in whichever way that needs to occur.

- 'Chew things over' but in a methodical, healthy way that ultimately leads to progress and transformation.

When the GodJuice in Stomach Meridian is blocked or unbalanced, you can experience the following emotional issues:

- You go round and round in circles, stuck in a comfort zone even if it's suffocating or unhealthy, unable to move on, or actually get anywhere.

■ You assimilate other people's 'stuff' instead of recognizing your own ideas, emotions and thoughts.

■ Your sense of truth can become compromised by your desire to keep things the way they are, and remain 'comfortable,' at any cost.

■ You lie to yourself about what you're really feeling or experiencing, especially if it's something negative. For example, you might lie about the negative consequences of your own, or other people's actions, or you might find yourself making excuses about the negative impact your desires or beliefs are having on your physical and mental health.

■ Both your general sense of trust, along with your trust in God, will disappear and you start worrying, agonizing and obsessing over even the most minor aspects of your day-to-day life. Obsessively worrying over the more minor and mundane aspects of life uses up so much energy, that there is precious little left over for loftier aspirations or big decisions.

■ You'll literally 'feel sick to your stomach' because of an emotional issue or disturbance you're experiencing.

■ Eating becomes fraught with difficulties and challenges: you'll comfort eat, overeat, binge eat, eat things that aren't good for you, or eat at times when you don't need to eat. Or, you might try to severely curtail your eating in an attempt to feel that you're really still in control.

■ You can feel as though you have a big emotional hole to fill, and a deep sense of unease and emptiness that no amount of food can satisfy.

And the following physical issues:

■ All manner of stomach issues, including poor digestion, acid indigestion and stomach ulcers

■ Cysts (both in the ovaries and in the breasts)

■ Fibroids

■ Swelling, particularly a swollen belly

■ Edema (water retention)

■ Mucus

- Weak muscles

- Metabolic disorders

- Macular degeneration

- Detached retinas

- Twitching eyes

- Stomach pain

- Sinusitis, and other sinus-related issues

- Ovary problems

- Hormone issues (particularly for females)

> *Spleen Meridian - Emotional energy when unbalanced: either too much compassion for others, and too little for the self, or too little compassion for others and too much for the self, or too little compassion for anyone and unable to accept and internalize others' ideas, feelings, or needs. Emotional energy when balanced: compassionate and caring, fair and generous with others, but not at the expense of the self and able to assimilate and respond to 'outside' information.*

Spleen

Out of all of the meridians in the body, Spleen energy is the most associated with feelings of happiness and joy. When you get stressed out, the first thing that goes out the window is your *joie de vivre*. Energetically-speaking, all the energy in all the meridians can get severely depleted and weakened by chronic stress, but the one that takes the biggest hit is Spleen Meridian.

That's because, together with the Triple Warmer Meridian, Spleen Meridian is responsible for running our immune system. Where Triple Warmer mobilizes the body's energies to respond to a perceived threat or danger, Spleen tries to keep you healthy by keeping you happy, full of vitality and joy.

In an emergency (i.e., whenever you get stressed out by something), Triple Warmer can pull energy away from all the meridians except the Heart to fuel it's 'flight or fight' response - and the first meridian it takes energy from is Spleen.

When the GodJuice in Spleen is flowing well you:

- Can easily metabolize your food, energy, knowledge and learning.

- Can digest things properly, in both the physical and mental realms, without experiencing any negative reactions.

- Can integrate new information and react appropriately to the things you're being told, along with the things that you're learning, instead of blanking the new information and blocking it out.

- Have a lot of healthy compassionate energy available, both for yourself and for others.

- Can more easily connect to your deeper self, your 'inner child,' and your sense of intuition.

When the GodJuice in Spleen Meridian is blocked or unbalanced, you can experience the following emotional issues:

- You find it hard to nurture yourself, and others, appropriately.

- Your ability to empathize with others is impaired.

- You can't stand up for yourself appropriately OR you can't take anyone else's view or opinion into account.

- You're more susceptible to developing a number of emotional disorders and issues, including: bipolar, schizophrenia, ADD / ADHD, and any personality disorder or condition characterized by a lack of, or unhealthy, empathy.

And the following physical issues:

- Autoimmune diseases including Fibromyalgia and Chronic Fatigue Syndrome

- Excessive, easy bruising

- Nosebleeds

- Varicose veins

- Any problems keeping the blood in the veins, arteries and blood vessels

- Diabetes

- Hypoglycemia

- Pancreas / blood sugar problems

- Allergies

- Immunodeficiency

- Issues related to pregnancy

- Hemorrhaging

- Blood clots

- General swelling and inflammation

- Issues with tear ducts

- Neuropathy (sore feet)

- Osteoporosis (if hormone-related)

- Anything on the heel

- Fasciitis

- Infections

- Depression

- Learning disorders, including ADHD

What Weakens Your Spleen Energy?

As you can see, weak Spleen energy is a major factor in so many of the most challenging and widespread illnesses and issues facing us in our modern world. Once you identify what might be making it so weak, you can start talking to God about turning things around. All of the following things could be wiping your Spleen energy out:

- Environmental pollution

- Unhealthy food and food additives

- Heavy-duty stress

- Electromagnetic energy (think PCs, mobiles, Wi-Fi, microwaves)

- Negative emotions

- Angry / critical / selfish / demanding people

- Not enough or too much compassion for ourselves, or others

- Ingratitude

- One-off shocks or traumatic experiences, including difficult births

Heart Meridian - *Emotional energy when unbalanced: heartache or a broken heart. Emotional energy when balanced: love, seeing the good in the self and others.*

Heart

The Heart Meridian is unique, inasmuch as it's the only place that the Triple Warmer Meridian can't take energy from.

When the GodJuice in the Heart Meridian is flowing well, you:

- Can still give, care and love, even in the face of stressful circumstances and enormously difficult challenges.

- Retain your fundamental belief in God's goodness, and you continue to look for - and to find - the good in yourself and in others, even if you've been through a lot yourself.

- Believe in your unique, God-given ability to build the world, and you're motivated to search for, and to find, the silver lining in even your most difficult circumstances.

- Have a strong sense of quiet optimism and spiritual resilience.

- Can feel and demonstrate love to yourself and to others, despite your own hardships.

When the GodJuice in Heart Meridian is blocked or unbalanced, you can experience the following emotional issues:

■ You carry around a profound sense of bitterness, hurt, rejection and mistrust. You become cynical about yourself, people in general and God.

■ Your ability to love can get buried under the huge defenses you throw up to keep your heart 'safe,' leaving you even more vulnerable to heartache, heartbreak, disappointment and hurt.

■ You try to protect yourself by keeping others at a distance, and train yourself to see the flaws in others, expecting the worst from people and the world to avoid having your heart broken again.

And the following physical issues:

■ Angina

■ Insomnia

■ Chest pains

■ Bleeding gums

■ Too hot / too cold

■ Blood pressure issues

■ Heart issues

■ Dizziness

■ Eczema

■ Circulation issues

> *Small Intestine Meridian - Emotional energy when unbalanced: pulled all over the place, confusion and inability to make decisions. Emotional energy when balanced: can act decisively and know what you want.*

Small Intestine

Energetically, Small Intestine Meridian is engaged in the job of absorption and discernment. It absorbs food, information, impressions and nutrients, etc., and then decides what needs to be kept and put to good use, and what needs to be discarded.

Small Intestine is the energy of clarification: everything you absorb into yourself will pass through the energy of the Small Intestine, physically and metaphorically speaking, where it will be thoroughly checked out, checked into, classified, and then dealt with accordingly.

When the GodJuice in the Small Intestine Meridian is flowing well, you:

- Can act decisively and make decisions quickly, without unnecessary dithering and procrastination.

- Can develop a deep, profound understanding and wisdom.

- Grasp even complicated issues and material easily, and can quickly break them down into their component parts, enabling you to make informed decisions.

When the GodJuice in Small Intestine Meridian is blocked or unbalanced, you can experience the following emotional issues:

- Even small decisions become agonizing, never-ending discussions, where it seems impossible to find the clarity required to make the correct choice.

- You can feel pulled all over the place, uncertain about what you want, what you need, or what the right decision should be.

- You frequently try to get other people involved in making your decisions for you, but each additional opinion only serves to further confuse matters and muddy the waters even more.

- Instead of having clarity and confidence, you feel confused and wracked with anxiety.

- You often start to panic when you need to make a quick decision about an important matter.

- Your decision-making process is often impulsive, rash and reactive.

And the following physical issues:

- Knee pain (over the tops of the knees)

- Weak thighs and legs

- Abdominal issues

- Beer bellies

- Ear problems

- Tinnitus

- Heart problems

> *Bladder Meridian - Emotional energy when unbalanced: fearful of the outside world, despairing, pessimistic. Emotional energy when balanced: strong belief in God's goodness, optimistic, trusting, courageous.*

Bladder

Bladder Meridian is the longest energy meridian you have, traveling down the length of your spine, from the crown of your head to the tips of your toes. Given its length, and close association with the spine, it should be of little surprise to learn that Bladder Meridian governs the nervous system.

When the GodJuice in Bladder Meridian is flowing well, you:

- Have a healthy, strong nervous system.

- Have the courage you need to move forward, the belief that things can improve and the will to change your life for the better.

- Have a strong sense of trust that whatever situation you're in right now, even if it's very challenging or difficult, it's somehow for your good, and your problems won't go on forever.

- Can easily buy into the idea that God has a solution waiting for you - even if you currently can't even begin to fathom what it might be - which can prevent you from sliding into despair, when you hit a tough patch.

When the GodJuice in Bladder Meridian is blocked or unbalanced, you can experience the following emotional issues:

- You can become very fearful and scared about what's going to be.

- You can get overwhelmed by problems, because you can't see any way of solving them.

- You can lose hope that the future is going to be any different or better, which can cause you to fall into a dark pit of futility and despair and contribute to feelings of depression.

- The outside world can become a dark, foreboding, and scary place.

- The fear of 'what will be?' can become overwhelming, particularly if you're going through a rough patch.

And the following physical issues:

- Headaches at the back of the head, or forehead

- Neuropathy (sore feet)

- Nervous system issues

- Poor hair growth

- Swollen ankles

- Bladder problems: urinary tract problems

- All sorts of back and shoulder pains

- Arthritis

- Rheumatism

- Bursitis

- Turned-in feet: foot and ankle problems, bunions, flat feet, fallen arches, etc.

- Feeling off-balance

- Hard to walk

- Feeling despairing, pessimistic and suspicious of everything and everyone

> *Kidney Meridian - Emotional energy when unbalanced: loneliness, ashamed of the self, traumatized, 'frozen,' existential angst. Emotional energy when balanced: deep acceptance of the self, strong, healthy connections to others, strong connection to God.*

Kidney

Kidney Meridian is the deepest meridian there is, and traditional Chinese medicine considers it to be the primary storehouse of the body's energy.

When you get a good start in life - however you care to define that - the GodJuice in your Kidney Meridian will usually be strong and vibrant. When you have a less-than-ideal start, from either the nature or nurture perspective, Kidney Meridian energy is usually one of the first places that starts to deplete, often leaving you feeling exhausted, and somehow lacking the will to continue.

Kidney Meridian deals with detoxification: it moves out the poisonous stuff that the body and soul no longer needs. When you become overwhelmed with emotional and physical toxins, this weakens your Kidney Meridian, making it much harder for it to do its 'clean-up' job. This can create a vicious cycle, where the toxins start to back up, weakening your Kidney Meridian still further, and reducing the amount of GodJuice available to deal with any toxic buildup.

Two of the most powerfully destructive 'toxic' emotions are fear and shame. If they aren't recognized, acknowledged and dealt with, they can overwhelm and seriously weaken Kidney Meridian, especially if they've been building up over time, or from childhood, without ever really being cleaned out of your system.

When the GodJuice in Kidney Meridian is flowing well, you:

- Feel vibrant, full of ideas, enthusiastic about life and very motivated to create, do, build and learn.

- Can develop strong visions of how good things could be.

- Become committed to searching for, and finding, the truth.

- Have loads of energy, and an infectious enthusiasm that enables you to easily inspire others to join you in your quest to change the world for the better.

- Can fully embrace the lessons of the past, while still being willing and able to start afresh and renew yourself.

When the GodJuice in Kidney Meridian is blocked or unbalanced, you can experience the following emotional issues:

- You can get 'stuck' in the past, or in events that happened long ago, or in old family sagas or patterns, unable to move forward.

- You can feel overwhelmed by very deeply-held (and often completely subconscious) feelings of toxic shame and guilt.

- You lose your *joie de vivre,* and in severe cases you can feel like you've lost your will to live.

- You feel exhausted, tired and sapped of your most basic life force.

- You can feel very defensive, and be very wary of discussing anything too personal or 'deep.'

And the following physical issues:

- Infertility and impotence

- Bone issues

- Weak eyesight and vision problems

- Lower backache

- Ears: ear infections, issues affecting balance and the inner ear

- Poor libido

- General health of teeth and gums

- Osteoporosis (bone-related)

- Throat problems

- Prostrate issues

- Knee pain

- Swollen / weak ankles or legs

- Sweaty feet

> *Circulation-Sex Meridian - Emotional energy when unbalanced: frustrated by 'over choice,' too many demands, ignoring their own deepest emotional needs, commitment-phobic. Emotional energy when balanced: has healthy priorities, recognizes and responds to their emotional needs, committed.*

Circulation-Sex

Circulation-Sex regulates systems in the body, as opposed to a particular organ. As the name suggests, the two main 'systems' being regulated by the energy in this meridian are the body's circulation, and its hormones.

When the GodJuice in Circulation-Sex Meridian is flowing well, you:

- Are full of energy, enthusiasm and joy, and you're the life-and-soul of the party.

- Find it very easy to act generous and caring.

- Can express yourself honestly and easily, and can form close, satisfying and healthy friendships.

- Feel at home in the world, liked and loved.

- Enjoy relationships that are characterized by acceptance, an easy and uncomplicated give-and-take of feelings, experiences and ideas, and a sense of love and mutual support that doesn't suffocate or squash anyone.

When the GodJuice in Circulation-Sex Meridian is blocked or unbalanced, you can experience the following emotional issues:

- You can find yourself feeling 'disconnected' and out of it.

- Your connection to your own sense of self becomes weak, making it difficult for you to know who, or what to trust, which can impact your ability to form fulfilling and honest relationships with others.

- You often feel confused, anxious and unsure about yourself, other people, and everything else, leading to situations where you're by turns too clingy, or too aloof and distant.

- You find it hard to commit to, and trust others.

- You can 'burn out' easily, if the energy and caring you continually put out into the world isn't recycled back to you.

- You can end up being surrounded by people who are struggling to commit to, trust, or deeply love others, leading to a proliferation of dysfunctional, complicated relationships.

- You can be prone to sudden mood changes, which only add to your confusion about who you really are, what you really want, and who (and what) is really good for you.

And the following physical issues:

- Hormonal issues

- Weak or cold legs

- Sciatica

- Blood pressure

- Cellulite

- Breast and nipple soreness or pain; production of breast milk

- Sexual problems

- Carpal tunnel

- Prostrate issues

- Impotence

- Sacrum issues

- Swollen armpits

- Sore glute muscles

> *Triple Warmer Meridian - Emotional energy when unbalanced: heavy-duty stress, the 'fight / flight / freeze' response, aka 'I'm taking control, here, and looking after Number 1.' The Triple Warmer Meridian's main emotions are primal fear and self-preservation. Nothing can kill our joy and our connection to God as fast and as effectively as a rampaging Triple Warmer. Emotional energy when balanced: feeling safe and secure, humbly trusting God's goodness.*

Triple Warmer

Triple Warmer, like Circulation-Sex, deals with a system, rather than a particular organ. Triple Warmer is probably the single most important meridian to get into balance, as it holds the energetic key to conquering your negative emotions and bad character traits. Here's how:

Energetically, the Triple Warmer Meridian is meant to work in tandem with the Spleen Meridian, as the second arm of your immune system. Where Spleen tries to keep you healthy by making you feel good, Triple Warmer tries to keep you healthy either by blasting any suspected 'threat' to pieces, or by running away from it (the infamous 'fight or flight response').

Whether it's a flu virus, a poisonous foodstuff, or an aggressive would-be assailant, Triple Warmer has the job of sizing up the potential threat or danger to the self (i.e., you) and then deciding whether it's better for you to try to fight your way out of the problem, or just run away from it.

If you get a virus, for example, Triple Warmer will react with a 'fight' response - your body's temperature will shoot way up to try and burn the virus out of your system, which you'll recognize as 'running a fever.'

If someone jumps out of the bushes at you, Triple Warmer will usually react - instantaneously - by giving you the strong impulse to run away as fast as you can, which is the classic 'flight' response.

Given the lifesaving nature of its work, the Triple Warmer Meridian has the ability to conscript energy from every meridian in the body, except the heart, to fuel your 'fight or flight' reflex. When Triple Warmer pulls energy away from the other meridians in the body, these other meridians are then temporarily weakened and unable to fulfill their proper energetic roles.

If your Triple Warmer was only being tripped off once or twice a day, it wouldn't matter so much. But modern life is so stressful, and apparently so full of potential threats and dangers, that most people's Triple Warmers are permanently switched on today, and reacting to perceived 'threats' 24/7.

The consequences of an over-reactive Triple Warmer

This has a number of consequences: When you go into Triple Warmer-induced 'fight' mode, that usually means that you're about to get overwhelmed by feelings of rage or anger. By contrast, when you go into 'flight' mode, you usually feel overwhelmed by strong feelings of fear or panic. When you fail to act on either of these 'fight or flight' impulses (because deep down, you know that you actually can't just punch your boss in the face, or run away from the social event where you've been cornered by the town letch) - then you can start to feel overwhelmed and hysterical. If this happens a lot, you can make a subconscious decision to kind of switch off from your feelings, and go emotionally 'numb,' as a coping strategy to help you deal with continually feeling overwhelmed by strong, negative emotions.

None of these things are helpful, from a spiritual, emotional or physical perspective.

Even if you're someone who usually tries to keep a lid on your negative emotions and your stress response, you may well find that even with your best efforts to stay calm, something very small and insignificant can happen that'll cause you to erupt in fury. Energetically, Triple Warmer is behind that response. It wants you to release all the immense emotional energy that you've been quietly building up while you're under stress, and it's pulling your strings so that you have a rage fit, instead of having a heart attack.

Triple Warmer depletes your Spleen energy

When you get stressed, the first place that Triple Warmer takes energy from is your Spleen Meridian, which governs your joy and ability to digest and metabolize food and knowledge, amongst other things. Chronically weak Spleen energy can mean that people lack *joie de vivre,* and can feel sad and depressed. Also, when you can't properly metabolize your food, and break it down into elements that your body can use, you can become intolerant or allergic to that food, or substance.

It only takes one allergic response for Triple Warmer to place that food, or allergen, firmly on its list of 'threats,' and from that point on, it will up the ante, and up the physical response you have to it. This is why even mild allergies can become bigger problems over time, if Triple Warmer isn't taught to back down.

If your birth or childhood was characterized by fear and stress, for whatever reasons, then it's almost guaranteed that your Triple Warmer will be turned on, and overreacting, way too much of the time. When this happens, it can literally change your whole demeanor, personality, and outlook on life.

Triple Warmer 'steals' the energy and the GodJuice from your other meridians

The energy and GodJuice that Triple Warmer steals from the other meridians when it mounts its 'fight or flight' response severely depletes your available emotional resources. Nine times out of ten, those resources could be put to much better use, helping you to have a much happier, healthier, more enjoyable and fulfilling life.

If Triple Warmer is taking energy from your Large Intestine Meridian, for instance, which governs issues involving holding on and releasing, you could start to develop some serious control issues. If Triple Warmer instead decides to steal some juice from your Gallbladder Meridian, which governs tolerance and judgment, you could start to judge others very harshly, leading to you developing feelings of rage, hatred, anger and intense dislike.

Let's take one more example: If Triple Warmer takes energy from your Bladder Meridian, which governs hope and optimism amongst other things, then it makes it much more likely that you could fall into feelings of pessimism and despair.

Triple Warmer maintains your habits

Triple Warmer also maintains our physical and mental habits. If you find yourself going into the 'same old routine' - reacting with the same words, the same hissy fit or the same sense of despair and depression - Triple Warmer is definitely at play, keeping you trapped in a negative pattern of energy that you probably desperately wish you could break out of. (The good news is: you can! In the Appendix on working with meridians, I'll give you a whole bunch of ways you can train Triple Warmer to start behaving better.)

And it's doing the same with your negative physical habits too; encouraging you to reach for the Scotch when you've had a hard day, or to reach for the cigarettes when you're stressed, or to reach for the chocolate when you're lonely, etc.

Now that we've got all the heavy stuff about Triple Warmer out of the way, you should know that there's a great many things you can do to take control of your Triple Warmer. Out of all the meridians, Triple Warmer responds the fastest to your intentions and conscious mind. It really acts very similarly to a small, hysterical child: if you take the time to reassure your Triple Warmer that you're actually OK, and to tell it that God is looking after you, it can start to calm down very fast.

So the main message you (and all of us...) need to give your Triple Warmer is:

> *'All is well. God is in control and it's all*
> *for my good. It's safe to let go.'*

Energetically, there are a number of things you can do to 'sedate' the energy in Triple Warmer, which forces it to give back stolen energy from other parts of the body, and I'll cover that stuff in detail in Appendix 1, at the back of the book.

When the GodJuice in Triple Warmer Meridian is blocked or unbalanced, you can experience the following issues:

- Feeling overwhelmed, panicked, anxious, angry, embarrassed or fearful

- Extreme shifts in temperature

- Sweating

- Autoimmune illnesses including asthma, hives

- Bipolar conditions

- Long-term depression

- Personality disorders

- Adrenal exhaustion

- Thyroid problems

- Hormonal problems, PMS

- Hysteria, hyperventilation, chattering teeth, chills, shaking, etc.

- MS

- Fever

- Emotional shock and trauma

- Menopause, hot flashes

- Weight problems

- Diabetes

- Allergies

> *Gallbladder Meridian - Emotional energy when unbalanced: anger at others, very judgmental and critical, unforgiving and demanding. Emotional energy when balanced: kind, merciful, tolerant and forgiving with healthy assertiveness.*

Gallbladder

Gallbladder governs the spectrum of emotions from tolerance to harsh judgment. It runs down both sides of your body, and is often involved in any 'one-sided' physical health issues you might have.

When the GodJuice in the Gallbladder Meridian is flowing well, you:

- Are tolerant of, and patient with others, which means that you try to judge them favorably and see them with a good eye.

- Have the self-confidence to act decisively, without treading on other people's toes in the process.

- Have the energy and courage you need to confront whatever needs confronting, to address it appropriately and fairly, to move forward in life and away from whatever suffocating or limiting role or circumstance you find yourself in.

When the GodJuice in Gallbladder Meridian is blocked or unbalanced, you can experience the following emotional issues:

- You struggle to control your feelings of harsh criticism, judgment and anger against other people.

- You have zero tolerance of errors and mistakes, zero patience when things aren't done as you'd like them to be, or delivered on time, and you don't hesitate to speak harshly, critically and forcefully against other people.

- Your relationships with other people can become tense, fragile and strained, marred by fits of jealousy and rage, inflexible intolerance, criticism and blame.

- If your feelings of anger and resentment towards other people aren't expressed but are pushed down, you can experience smoldering resentment, hatred and an inability to forgive and move on.

- You can behave passive-aggressively, often experiencing sullen moods and intense feelings of frustration at objects, things and situations (instead of at the people who are really making you angry).

- You feel unable to really listen, change, confront, or discuss anything of substance.

And the following physical issues:

- TMJ: jaw pain

- One-sided headaches (temple headaches)

- Migraines

- Grinding teeth

- Pain on side of eyes

- Swollen ankles

- Sciatica

- Gallstones

- Addicted to sedatives (alcohol, pills, marijuana)

- Addicted to stimulants (coffee, sugar, cigarettes)

- High blood pressure

- Hip problems

- Shingles

Liver Meridian - Emotional energy when unbalanced: 'beating ourselves up,' hypercritical of the self, feelings of guilt. Emotional energy when balanced: positive feelings about the self, self-forgiveness and acceptance, able to nurture and care for the self.

Liver

Liver Meridian governs pressure buildup and direction, both energetically and physically. It sends powerful amounts of energy and blood around your body, and confronts poisons and challenges to your spiritual and physical health, in an effort to detox you.

Emotionally, Liver energy can also really move mountains, and is very responsive to the power of the mind - both for good and for bad.

When the GodJuice in the Liver Meridian is flowing well, you:

- Can be focused, assertive, truthful and confident - but not at anybody else's expense.

- Have clarity about what needs to happen, and when, and how, but this will come along with a big dose of kindness and a profound understanding that different people do different things in different ways.

- Look for ways to encourage others to make the best use of their innate, God-given talents and abilities, instead of demanding that people bend to your will, your way, or your vision.

- Cut yourself, and other people, a lot of slack, and you understand that true, lasting success often requires a great deal of trial and error.

- Get things done, and you aren't afraid to try new things and grow in different directions.

■ Enjoy being yourself, and you don't feel threatened by differences. You have enough inner confidence to stand out from the crowd, or to swim against the tide, if that's the path you need to go on, and you will give everything you have to a cause, mission or job you believe in.

When the GodJuice in Liver Meridian is blocked or unbalanced, you can experience the following emotional issues:

■ You start beating yourself up a lot - about everything - and you can start to feel frustrated and angry with yourself for not doing things differently, or better, or like so-and-so.

■ You blame yourself mercilessly whenever something goes wrong, and can judge yourself very harshly.

■ You feel guilty for being 'flawed you,' instead of Mr. or Ms. Perfect.

■ You start to view your quirks and eccentricities as problematic.

■ You can become a fierce believer in doing things 'by the book,' and start to feel threatened when others start to develop more of an individual streak, or begin to pull away from your 'normal,' accepted way of doing things.

■ You can easily get lost 'in the process'; you can be so busy trying to 'make things happen' that you can lose sight of what you're actually doing it all for.

■ You struggle to be patient with yourself and others, because you can clearly see where you want to get to (or what you want others to do) - but you can't seem to make it happen.

■ You can find it hard to wake up without a coffee or some other stimulant, and / or you frequently turn to pills, alcohols or some other sedative to help you 'slow down.'

And the following physical issues:

■ Eyes: teary eyes, 'sun is too bright' issues, blurry vision, spots before the eyes

■ Cataracts, astigmatism

■ Candida

- Thick, yellow toenails

- Fungus issues

- General toxicity

- Tendency to drink too much (coffee, alcohol)

- Hypertension

- Tightness in the chest and / or upper back

- PMS

- Jaundice

- Menopause issues

- Hepatitis

- Low sperm count

> **Lung Meridian** - *Emotional energy when unbalanced: profound sadness and grief, yearning, unwillingness to get emotionally involved with others, aloof. Emotional energy when balanced: belief in God's goodness, renewal, excitement, an ability to let go and move on, ability to connect to others at the deepest levels.*

Lungs

The Lung Meridian contains the last energy before death - it's literally the last 'breath' that you'll take. Fittingly, Lung energy is about evaluation, completion and closure.

When the GodJuice in the Lung Meridian is flowing well, you:

- Have high ethical standards, clarity, and a humble and even reverent, respect for others.

- Have a lot of deep insight and thoughtfulness.

- Can deal with 'ends' and conclusions and 'partings' without getting overwhelmed by grief and sadness.

- Have a profound awareness that you are here to do a job, which means that you efficiently and shrewdly measure everything against this backdrop of achieving the ultimate goal of life.

- Recognize that 'ends' have to happen for 'beginnings' to start, and self-renewal comes easily and often to you.

- Can easily let go of things that you no longer require, or need, while still being profoundly grateful for having had the thing, person or experience in your life, in the first place.

- Are grateful for even the small things in life, (like taking a breath of fresh air) and you'll be aware of what's really important and worthwhile.

- Stay focused on your higher goals, and you'll actively pursue your more spiritual dimension.

- Inspire others to evaluate and consider their path in life, and to ponder what happens 'after the last breath' has been taken.

- Aren't scared of being alone, and you'll use your inevitable periods of 'aloneness' for introspection, re-evaluation, prayer and inner growth.

When the GodJuice in Lung Meridian is blocked or unbalanced, you can experience the following emotional issues:

- You can easily become gloomy, sad and detached from others, because it's all going to end, anyway, so what's the point in trying to do anything, or in opening yourself up to anyone, or in loving someone else?

- You can find yourself 'holding your breath,' waiting for bad things to happen.

- You can become very disillusioned with life, and find yourself mechanically going through the motions, instead of living life to the full.

- The idea of having 'fun,' or breaking the rules, or doing things differently and spontaneously becomes anathema to you.

- You can get stuck on, or left behind in, your massive disappointments, unable to let go of them and move on in your life.

- You can become a stickler for rules, order, and dry, boring, predictability, and you can get very upset when someone or something disrupts your formality and routine, however much it may actually be suffocating you.

- You find it very hard to cope when structure disappears from your life.

- Your 'aloneness' can quickly turn into a profound sense of loneliness, pessimism and gloom.

And the following physical issues:

- Can't breathe properly

- Tuberculosis

- Pneumonia

- Shortness of breath

- Insomnia (in the early morning)

- Skin problems: itching

- Frozen shoulder: problems with the shoulder cap

- Colds, coughs

- Flu

- Bronchitis

> *Large Intestine Meridian - Emotional energy when unbalanced: control-freak, a need to be in control even when it's damaging the self and others. Emotional energy when balanced: surrenders control; can let go of outmoded, unneeded, or toxic things.*

Large Intestine

You can sum up the energy of Large Intestine like this: It's all about the ability to let go. Large Intestine energy is also associated with maintaining high standards, acting ethically and with integrity, playing by the rules, and sticking to the letter of the law.

When the GodJuice in the Large Intestine Meridian is flowing well, you:

- Still make your best efforts to act appropriately, to succeed, and to do the right thing, but you'll also find it easy to let go and to hand ultimate control back to God.

- Understand that while you have to make an effort, and to strive to do your best, the final outcome is not up to you: it's up to God.

- Are happy with your lot in life, which means you can be flexible, relaxed and accepting, even when life isn't going the way you planned, and even when you're facing some very difficult challenges.

- Give out a lot of 'light,' even in the middle of the darkness, and people are still attracted to you and enjoy your company.

When the GodJuice in Large Intestine Meridian is blocked or unbalanced, you can experience the following emotional issues:

- Your ability to 'let go' becomes blocked, and you can develop pedantic control-freak tendencies.

- You'll still want to do the right thing, but you get bogged down in all the rules and externals, which can prevent you from accessing the more important inner dimension.

- You can become controlled by your 'control freak' energy, becoming worried, anxious and depressed when even the smallest detail doesn't go to plan.

- You start to develop an unhealthy desire for things to be 'perfect.'

- You can become inflexible, arrogant and rigid, and find it very difficult to let go of what you want, or what you think - even when you can see it's harming you, in some way.

And the following physical issues:

- Digestion issues

- Colonic disorders

- Constipation / Diarrhea

- Hemorrhoids

- Hip problems

- Herpes

- Lower back pain

- Nose problems

- Mineral deficiencies

- Toothaches

- Cellulite (on the thighs)

What do I do next?

In the next chapter, we'll go into more detail about how to start pulling all the different parts of your personal health puzzle together.

If you already know what your physical issues are, an easy way to start is to check to see what meridian, or meridians they could be associated with, using the easy-to-use quick reference guide on page 185.

Also, if you already know what your physical issues are, an easy way to start is to check to see what meridian, or meridians, they could be associated with, using the following easy-to-use quick reference guide below. Alternatively, if you already know that you have a particular emotional issue or challenge, hopefully you'll be heartened to learn that it's not necessarily hardwired into your psyche, but could well be the result of an energetic imbalance in your body's meridians.

Once the energy is unblocked and strengthened in a particular meridian, the emotional and spiritual issue will also start to move by itself, even if no additional conscious thought is given to it.

In Appendix 1 at the back of the book, you'll find a brief guide describing how to trace, sedate and strengthen the 12 main energy meridians, and in many instances, these basic acupressure tools could be all you need to get things moving for you, especially if you're also putting God in the picture.

You don't need to be an expert in Energy Medicine, acupressure, applied kinesiology, or even in praying to get the techniques in this book to work for you. You just need to be willing to give things a try, to put God in the picture, and to grasp the basic concept that the best, fastest and most efficient approach to resolving your health and emotional issues is to work on them from both angles, body and soul, together.

RECAP

Central Meridian - Emotional energy when unbalanced: feeling vulnerable or 'lacking.' Emotional energy when balanced: feeling grounded, confident and secure.

Governing Meridian - Emotional energy when unbalanced: unable to move forward, 'no backbone.' Emotional energy when balanced: 'can-do ability,' having the courage to move on, overcome problems and try new things.

Stomach Meridian - Emotional energy when unbalanced: anxiety, pessimism and extreme worry about day-to-day problems and needs. Emotional energy when balanced: trust that everything will turn out OK, calm, serene and with a strong belief in God's goodness.

Spleen Meridian - Emotional energy when unbalanced: either too much compassion for others and too little for the self, or too little compassion for others and too much for the self, or too little compassion for anyone and being unable to accept and internalize others' ideas, feelings, or needs. Emotional energy when balanced: compassionate and caring, fair and generous with others but not at the expense of the self and able to assimilate and respond to 'outside' information.

Heart Meridian - Emotional energy when unbalanced: heartache or a broken heart. Emotional energy when balanced: love, seeing the good in the self and others.

Small Intestine Meridian - Emotional energy when unbalanced: pulled all over the place, confusion and inability to make decisions. Emotional energy when balanced: can act decisively and know what you want.

Bladder Meridian - Emotional energy when unbalanced: fearful of the outside world, despairing, pessimistic. Emotional energy when balanced: strong belief in God's goodness, optimistic, trusting and courageous.

Kidney Meridian - Emotional energy when unbalanced: loneliness, ashamed of the self, traumatized, 'frozen,' with existential angst. Emotional energy when balanced: deep acceptance of the self, strong, healthy connections to others and strong connection to God.

Circulation-Sex Meridian - Emotional energy when unbalanced: frustrated by 'over choice,' too many demands, ignoring their own deepest emotional needs, commitment-phobic. Emotional energy when balanced: has healthy priorities, recognizes and responds to their emotional needs, committed.

Triple Warmer Meridian - Emotional energy when unbalanced: heavy-duty stress, the 'fight / flight / freeze' response, aka 'I'm taking control, here, and looking after Number 1.' The Triple Warmer's main emotions are primal fear and self-preservation. Nothing can kill our joy and our connection to God as fast and as effectively as a rampaging Triple Warmer. Emotional energy when balanced: feeling safe and secure, humbly trusting God's goodness.

Gallbladder Meridian - Emotional energy when unbalanced: anger at others, very judgmental and critical, unforgiving and demanding. Emotional energy when balanced: kind, merciful, tolerant and forgiving, with healthy assertiveness.

Liver Meridian - Emotional energy when unbalanced: 'beating ourselves up,' hypercritical of the self, feelings of guilt. Emotional energy when balanced: positive feelings about the self, self-forgiveness and acceptance, able to nurture and care for the self.

Lung Meridian - Emotional energy when unbalanced: profound sadness and grief, yearning, unwillingness to get emotionally involved with others, aloof. Emotional energy when balanced: belief in God's goodness, renewal, excitement, an ability to let go and move on, the ability to connect to others at the deepest levels.

Large Intestine Meridian - Emotional energy when unbalanced: control-freak, a need to be in control even when it's damaging the self and others. Emotional energy when balanced: surrenders control, can let go of outmoded, unneeded, or toxic things.

Chapter 8

Putting It Into Practice

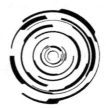

n this chapter, we're going to start pulling together everything you've learned so far and show you how applying the ideas in this book can lead to some real, tangible improvements in your emotional and physical health.

First, let's recap the three main reasons why you get sick. (Note: There's actually a fourth, and last, reason why you get sick, but it's an exception not a rule, so I'll tell you more about it in the last chapter.)

- **The first reason you get sick: your GodJuice is blocked or weak**

- **The second reason you get sick: you have emotionally-unhealthy habits**

- **The third reason you get sick: God is using your specific illness to achieve a specific outcome or change**

The 'Talk to God and Fix Your Health' Questionnaire in this chapter contains a number of diagnostic tools and exercises that will hopefully help you to start figuring out which of the three areas mentioned above should be your first port of call, to get your GodJuice unstuck and your energy flowing again.

Once you've gone through the Questionnaire, you'll be ready to try some of the practical ideas and techniques contained in the Appendixes in the back of the book, to help you get your physical energy and emotions unblocked easily, safely and quickly.

Diagnosing the root of the problem

This next bit takes a little time and a bit of honesty, but by the end of the process you should have a really clear picture of where your energy's blocked and why, and how that could be making you sick.

While it's very common to start over-analyzing your responses as you go through the Questionnaire, it'll work best if you keep your answers simple and spontaneous: just write down the very first thing that comes to mind.

If you find you're blanking or dithering over an answer, it could be because you've just stumbled upon some uncomfortable truth that on some level you're worried about acknowledging or accepting.

If that happens to you, don't sweat: just go and talk to God about it. When the time is right, He'll bring up whatever piece of knowledge or information or insight you need to move you on to the next part of your healing process.

The Three Rules of How NOT to Use This Section:

On no account should you do any of the following three things, as you go through this chapter:

1. Don't beat yourself up for not being able to do this 'right.'

2. Don't get too anxious about what might be lurking inside you (remember, the real you is ONLY good).

3. Don't get angry or frustrated that the process of getting real answers is taking a bit longer, or is a bit harder or more complicated, than you thought.

Your problems and issues didn't just magically appear overnight, and it's pretty unlikely that they're going to instantly vanish (although when you're working across all three levels of the problem, i.e., mind, body and soul - anything is possible).

If you stick to these rules, you should start to see certain things fall into place in your life, in a really neat way.

THE TALK TO GOD AND FIX YOUR HEALTH QUESTIONNAIRE

Part I: How Strong Is Your GodJuice?

Rate each of the following statements as follows:

0 - Almost never

1 - Sometimes

2 - Often

3 - Almost always

1. I believe in God.

2. I believe God is running the world, generally.

3. I believe God is directly behind everything that happens to me in life.

4. I believe that everything that happens to me will somehow turn around for the best.

5. I believe that God loves me.

6. I think about God.

7. I talk to God.

8. I don't just talk to God, I also try to listen to Him.

9. I'm prepared to put what God wants ahead of what I want.

10. If I knew 100% what God really wanted from me, I'd be willing to do it.

Add up your scores, and let's see where you're holding, Divine energy-wise:

0 - 10	=	**Critically weak**
11 - 15	=	**Weak**
16 - 20	=	Moderate
21 - 26	=	**Very strong**
27 - 30	=	**Impossible, as nobody's perfect**

If your score was weak or critically weak: You don't have enough GodJuice flowing through your system to keep you consistently happy and healthy, long-term, regardless of what else you might be doing to stay fit. Below, you'll find some instant 'quick fixes' that you can do to immediately boost your connection to God.

If your score was moderate: You have enough GodJuice to function reasonably well, especially if your scores in the other areas are strong, but there is definitely some room for improvement.

If your score was very strong: Keep doing what you're doing, you're definitely on the right path.

If your score was impossibly good: Either you need a little more work on your self-awareness and honesty, or you're the Messiah. I guess time will tell which one it is.

How to boost your GodJuice

Step 1: Check to see which statements you marked with a '0' - these are your main areas of work. (If you marked all the statements with a '0,' I'm amazed you got this far in the book. Maybe secretly, you actually believe in God a whole lot more than you're admitting to yourself?)

If you have no '0's, work with the '1's.

Step 2: Write down the statements you marked with a '0' (or a '1,' if you have no zeros).

Step 3: Talk to God about getting this specific area fixed, for at least five minutes, at least once.

Just doing the three steps outlined above, regardless of the outcome, will instantly connect you back to God, and start to boost your GodJuice.

"But I don't know what to say..."

If you don't know what to say when you're talking to God about strengthening the areas that you've identified as needing some work, try some of the following ideas to get your conversation started:

Statement: I believe in God

"God, that's exactly the problem! I don't believe in You. I'd love to think that You really do exist, and You really could solve all my problems for me, the way this crazy, naïve, lunatic is trying to tell me, but really? I can't. So God, if You really do exist, I need some convincing. Show me it's true! Show me You're real! Prove it..."

Statement: I believe God is running the world, generally

"It's like that book about the blind watchmaker. Sure, maybe You created the world all those years ago, but now? You're gone. You're out of the picture. You're 'up there,' and I'm 'down here,' and there's nothing connecting the two. I'm finding it really hard to believe that You're behind global warming, or terrorism, or the Dow Jones. But I'm willing to be convinced, so if You're really running the world, please show me, God. Show me really clearly, in a way that I can really get it."

Statement: I believe God is directly behind everything that happens to me in life

"You exist, I know that. Maybe I can even accept that You're making the grass grow, and the flowers bloom, and the birds migrate, and all that other stuff I watch on the Nature Channel. But when it comes to me and my life? God, I just can't see *You* in it. I can't feel You in it. Right now, I believe that there is one person responsible for my life: me. If that's wrong and You're really pulling the strings behind the scenes, I want to see how. I want to know that it's not just all random circumstance and chance, and that You really are in the picture."

Statement: I believe that everything that happens to me will somehow turn around for the best

"Please, how on earth am I meant to believe *that*? This lady has no idea how much bad stuff I've already had to deal with; how many things went wrong, or sour, how many times I've been hurt, let-down, disappointed and betrayed. How am I meant to believe *this,* for crying out loud? God, show me how that [really bad thing that happened to me 10 years ago] is 'for the best.' I'm really, really struggling to see it, especially as I'm still dealing with all the fallout."

Statement: I believe that God loves me

"God, if this is true, then why do You keep making me suffer? Why have I got all these issues? Why have I got all these problems? Why am I going through life feeling so unloved, alone and miserable? If You really love me, why haven't I got a ton of money / a great marriage / wonderful kids / my health / a fulfilling career / inner peace / big biceps / [your own particular complaint here]?

If You really do love me, why am I struggling so much, with so many things? Why aren't You giving me what I want?"

Statement: I think about God

"I don't know how thinking about God is meant to change anything in my life, or my health. How is just thinking about You meant to help me? What's this woman talking about? Is she seriously expecting me to think about You 24/7? That's not realistic, and it's not healthy. I'm not aspiring to be a monk or a spiritual ascetic. I don't get it. God, what does it mean, that I need to 'think about God'?"

Statement: I talk to God

"We both know only crazies talk to God: I see them on the street 'talking to God' all the time. I'm taking a big risk even trying this out for five minutes. So God, if You're really out there, show me You're listening. Show me why talking to You is going to help me fix my life, and specifically my health. Please give me some solid feedback...Give me some tangible sign that You're really hearing me..."

Statement: I don't just talk to God, I also try to listen to Him

"Now, what in the world is that meant to mean? How am I meant to be 'listening' to You, God? I don't get it. What does it even mean? How am I even meant to do that, exactly?"

(When you get the answer to these questions popping up in your head, don't ignore them or dismiss them - that's God, talking to you.)

Statement: I'm prepared to put what God wants ahead of what I want

"God, how can I agree to that statement? What if You want me to do something that I don't want to do? Or something that's not in my best interests? How can I even know what it is You actually want from me? You always want me to have the same things that I want me to have...don't You? And if not, then it would be really dumb to put what You want ahead of what I want. Why should I do it? What's in it, for me?"

Statement: If I knew 100% what God really wanted from me, I'd be willing to do it

"Man, that is a level, and I'm just not there. I don't know if anyone's really there (except the people who scored a straight '30' on this quiz...). How can I know what You really want from me? And how can I do it, especially if it's something hard, or uncomfortable, or painful, or challenging?

"I've got two main issues with this statement: First, I often don't have the first clue what You really want from me. Second, I don't know if I've got the guts or motivation to actually do it, even if I did know. Help me out, God. Give me the clarity and courage I need to really start making some changes for the better in my life, and to fulfill my potential."

Come clean, and be real

All these conversations are just examples, to get you started. You don't have to stick to them rigidly - and you don't even have to use them at all, if they don't speak to you. The point is, to be spontaneous, and to be honest, and to not censor yourself when you're talking to God. Come clean, as much as you can. God prefers your ugly truths much more than your beautiful lies.

If you get stuck, or struck dumb, refer back to the guidelines in Chapter 2, 'How to get your GodJuice humming'. You can also talk to God about helping you find the words to talk to Him. If you really want to get the conversation started it will happen, one way or another, so please don't get discouraged and give up.

The plain act of trying to talk to God - even if you are unable to say a single word - instantly connects your soul back to its Power source, boosts your GodJuice, and puts you back on the road to more happiness and better health.

The next place your energy can get blocked is your emotional health, and this will show up as an imbalance in one or more of the three foundations of emotional health. The following exercises will help you to identify where the imbalance may be.

HEALTHY COMPASSION

Rate each of the following statements as follows:

0 - Almost never

1 - Sometimes

2 - Often

3 - Almost always

1. If someone asks me for a favor, I do it.

2. I find it hard to spend time, money, or effort on myself.

3. I find it hard to see, or accept, someone else's point of view.

4. I look after 'Number One'.

5. I put other people's needs ahead of my own.

6. I feel other people's pain.

7. I find it easy to say 'no' to other people's requests.

8. I help other people out.

9. I hurt other people's feelings.

10. I'm motivated by self-interest.

If you scored between 21-30:

You probably tend to have too much, inappropriate compassion for others, and then wind up getting hurt by them. To stop that from happening, you need to put some clear boundaries in place. (You'll find some tips on how to do that in Chapter 6.)

If you scored between 10-20:

It looks like your compassion is pretty balanced! If you're a borderline score, you might want to read the rest of this section anyway, about how to fix unhealthy compassion, to learn more tips and tools for how you can keep things that way.

If you scored between 0-9:

You probably have a tendency to have too little compassion for everyone (including yourself). The following things will help you to start regaining balance:

How to Fix Unhealthy Compassion

1) Recognize The Problem

There are two main reasons why you're not treating other people with healthy compassion. Either:

- You didn't get enough healthy compassion yourself, so you have no idea how to replicate it.

OR

- Your Spleen energy is completely busted, and until you fix it, you haven't got enough 'compassionate juice' flowing around your system to treat anyone compassionately, including yourself.

2) Get God Involved

Take the problem back to God, discuss it with Him, and ask Him to help you resolve it.

3) Practice The Four Rules Of Healthy Compassion

Be warned, this is the hard part. It will probably take a lot of practice until responding in this way becomes second nature, so every time you manage to respond in the following way, celebrate it!

Don't get demoralized if this feels like pulling teeth, especially initially. When you hit a bad patch, or an obstacle, just take it back to God and tell Him what's going on. Sooner or later, the clouds will part and you'll find it much easier to respond with healthy compassion.

The Four Rules of Healthy Compassion:

1. Ask about the other person and / or their situation - as though you're really interested.

2. Listen attentively to their response - don't yawn, roll your eyes or cut them off mid-sentence.

3. Reflect what they just said back to them, so they know you really heard and understood them.

4. On no account blame them, criticize them, judge them, or start dishing out unsolicited advice. Your job is just to make the other person feel heard, cared for and loved.

I know, acting compassionately can be a real pain, can't it? But when you start to see how people begin to open up more around you, to trust you more and to enjoy your company more, you won't mind it so much anymore, I promise.

4) Strengthen Your Spleen Meridian

Boosting your GodJuice and following the steps outlined above to strengthen and balance your compassion will automatically start strengthening your Spleen Meridian too. See the Appendixes for practical tips on what you can do to strengthen your Spleen Meridian directly, using Energy Medicine techniques.

SENSIBLE ACCOUNTABILITY

Rate each of the following statements as follows:

0 - Almost never

1 - Sometimes

2 - Often

3 - Almost always

1. I apologize when I do something wrong.

2. I hate saying sorry.

3. I feel guilty.

4. I feel ashamed of my behavior.

5. When there's a problem, it's the other guy's fault.

6. When there's a problem, it's my fault.

7. I get emotional.

8. I make mistakes.

9. I feel bad when I do something wrong.

10. I act responsibly.

If you scored between 21-30:

Go back through your answers, and see if you can catch any inconsistencies. If you're scoring highly in this section that could mean that somewhere along the line, you might be making assumptions about yourself and your behavior that might not be true.

If you're still scoring on the high side once you've reevaluated your answers, you may be taking far too much responsibility for keeping other people happy in life, without realizing the toll it's taking on you.

If you scored between 10-20:

Your sense of accountability is pretty healthy. Carry on doing whatever it is you're doing!

If you scored between 0-9:

You probably don't spend a lot of time taking stock of your actions, and how they may be impacting other people (and yourself too).

That could be pointing to the fact that you have a tendency to not take enough responsibility for things.

Take heart, it's pretty easy to fix unbalanced accountability, once you know what's causing it. The next section tells you how.

How to Fix Unhealthy Accountability

1) Recognize the Problem

You're accountability can get out of whack in two distinct ways. Either:

- You're taking too much responsibility, and you feel guilt-ridden, ashamed and 'to blame' too much of the time.

OR

- You don't take enough responsibility (probably as a defense mechanism to being overly criticized, shamed or blamed as a child).

2) Get God Involved and Ask For Help

If you get stuck or blocked at any point in the clean-up process, just rev up your GodJuice, and ask God for help.

3) Practice Developing Your Own Voice of Reason, Using the Following Guidelines:

Voice of Reason Rule 1:

Remember nobody's perfect, and we all make mistakes sometimes.

<u>Voice of Reason Rule 2:</u>

Treat yourself at least as nicely as you treat other people.

<u>Voice of Reason Rule 3:</u>

Don't go to extremes - just look for the message. Don't beat yourself up, and don't let yourself off the hook.

4) Check To See If What You Think You're Doing 'Wrong' Is Included in the List of Five Big No-Nos

(You can find the Five Big No-Nos in Chapter 4.)

If it is, you need to apologize for what you did, and make a serious effort to try to change your behavior. If it isn't - forget about it.

5) Use the Tools in the 'Guide to Dissolving Your Emotional Blocks' (in Appendix 2) to Work on the Following Underlying Emotions

If your sense of accountability is unbalanced, the following underlying emotions usually have something to do with it.

- Guilt
- Toxic Shame
- Fear
- Overwhelm
- Self-Hatred

APPROPRIATE KINDNESSES

Rate each of the following statements as follows:

0 - Almost never

1 - Sometimes

2 - Often

3 - Almost always

1. When someone asks you for help, you should give it them.

2. You should put other people's needs ahead of your own.

3. I allow myself to get persuaded by others.

4. If I do someone a favor, I feel they owe me.

5. If someone does me a favor, I feel obliged to them.

6. I'm obliged to help others out.

7. I only do kindnesses when it suits me.

8. I know what's best for other people.

9. Saying 'no' makes me feel bad.

10. I enjoy being asked to do things for others.

If you scored between 21-30:

A high score in this section suggests that your kindnesses and favors often involve a big dose of reciprocation. Obligation, duty and 'doing the right thing' are probably big motivating factors for you.

If everyone is clear about what's going on, and what's being expected in return - great. If not, you're running a risk that your kindnesses could very easily cross the line into becoming 'controlling,' stressful and unhealthy - both for you, and for others.

If you scored between 10-20:

You do kindnesses for others in a healthy way, which means that you don't expect too much in return from other people; you can say 'no' when you need to and you enjoy the kindnesses you do.

If you scored between 0-9:

You may have been caught up in a whole load of manipulation, guilt and coercion in the past, and now you prefer to keep your kindnesses strictly to yourself.

That's understandable - but the person who's missing out the most in this situation is *you*. When you can choose to do healthy kindnesses for others with a full heart, it'll make you feel great.

How to Fix Unhealthy Kindness

1) Recognize the Problem

If you're genuinely choosing to do a kindness or favor for someone else (i.e., you WANT to do it) then it will fill you up, energize you and make you feel great.

If you're consistently being manipulated or coerced into putting other people's wishes ahead of your own (i.e., you or someone else is consistently telling you that you SHOULD do it) you'll feel exhausted, guilty, resentful, angry, frustrated, despairing and depressed.

Because this is usually occurring at the subconscious level, you often won't realize how much upset or stress these 'forced kindnesses' are causing you, as most of your negative emotions are being repressed.

If you have or have had a chronic health problem that hasn't responded to any other treatment, the chances are very high that it's rooted in 'unhealthy kindness.'

2) Get God Involved and Ask For Help

This applies to all issues, at all times. But it's particularly important when you're dealing with serious subconscious issues which can often be hard to reach, or resolve in more conventional ways.

God knows what your subconscious buttons are; He knows who and what is pressing them and He knows exactly what you need to do to unplug them to become happy and healthy again. Ask Him to clue you in!

3) Put Firm Boundaries In Place, Using The Following Three Rules (from Chapter 6):

Rule 1: Accept that not everyone is nice

Rule 2: Learn to trust your gut instincts

Rule 3: Walk away

4) Use the Tools in the 'Guide to Dissolving Your Emotional Blocks' (in Appendix 2) to Work on the Following Underlying Emotions

If your kindnesses are inappropriate, forced or missing, that's often linked to the following emotions:

- Anger
- Anxiety
- Beating yourself up
- Depression
- Despair
- Emptiness
- Fear
- Feeling 'out of control'
- Guilt
- Hatred
- Indecision
- Loneliness
- Nervousness
- Obsession (e.g., keep replaying conversations, etc., in your head)
- Panic

- Rage
- Resentment
- Self-hatred
- Shame
- Stress
- Worry

If an energy blockage, imbalance or weakness in a meridian is not dealt with, over time it can manifest as a *bona fide* emotional, mental or physical illness or issue.

Usually the physical problem only shows up in the first place because you've somehow got disconnected from the feeling, emotion or reaction that's causing the blockage. If you're not aware of the emotion that's causing the physical problem, how are you meant to identify it and get rid of the blockage?

That's where this section comes into its own, because as you've been learning nine times out of ten, God is only sending you the physical issue to show you the underlying problem, issue or emotion that you need to work on.

I've included a few different exercises and tools that you can do to try to tease out the information about what's really going on. If you do them, you should start to build up a fairly accurate picture of the energy and emotional dimension of your health; how they're linked and what meridians and emotions you need to make your priority for good health.

How to Use These Lists

Step 1: Circle the attributes that you feel most apply to you (and remember, these will change from day to day and week to week, as your energy, feelings and circumstances are constantly in a state of flux).

Step 2: Identify which meridian, or meridians, they're related to.

For the list of <u>Positive Attributes</u>, the ones you DIDN'T circle are the ones that probably need strengthening.

For the list of <u>Negative Attributes</u>, you will normally need to sedate, or unblock, the meridian associated with the words you circled.

(See the Basic Guide to Working with Your Energy Meridians, in Appendix 1, at the back of the book, for instructions on how to actually do that.)

Step 3: Try to identify any connections between specific illnesses and specific issues.

Identify which meridians keep coming up, as being weak, blocked or unbalanced in some way, then refer to the Quick Reference Tool: Meridians and their Associated Physical Issues, to see if anything starts to ring a bell for you.

EXERCISE 1: Circle the words that best describe how you generally feel (do this intuitively - circle whatever comes to mind without trying to analyze it):

Angry	Frustrated	Upset	Disappointed
Guilty	Switched-off	Numb	Happy
Satisfied	Filled-up	Empty	Blocked
Energized	Vengeful	Jealous	Competitive
Accepting	Judgmental	Fearful	Joyful
Safe	Overwhelmed	Capable	Judged
Right	Wrong	Successful	Failure
Loved	Loving	Exhausted	Friendly
Unfriendly	Relaxed	Stressed	Flexible
Rigid	Flowing	Stuck	Optimistic
Controlling	Worried	Upbeat	Kind
Selfish	Competent	Confident	Outgoing
Shy	Reserved	Quiet	Loud
Tired	Liked	Popular	Normal
Unusual	Outsider	Confused	Decisive
Unpopular	Real	Phony	Strong
Cynical			

Now, use the following lists of Positive and Negative Attributes and Emotions to identify where a specific emotion and / or energy meridian might be blocked.

Tip: Photocopy this page before you begin, so you can reuse this exercise again in the future.

Positive Attributes and Emotions

> *If you DIDN'T CIRCLE any of the following words in Exercise 1, that could be an indication that:*
> - *The energy flowing through the related meridian is weak, unbalanced or blocked.*
> - *You might be finding it hard to feel or express the following positive emotions and attributes:*

Attribute	Related meridian(s)
Accepting	Spleen, Heart, Liver
Capable	Liver, Spleen, Heart, Kidney
Competent	Liver, Spleen
Confident	Kidney, Spleen, Liver
Decisive	Small Intestine, Circulation-Sex
Energized	Spleen, Kidney
Filled-up	Large Intestine, Stomach
Flexible	Large Intestine, Heart
Flowing	Lungs, Large Intestine, Small Intestine
Friendly	Spleen, Kidney, Circulation-Sex, Lung, Heart
Happy	Spleen, Lungs, Liver, Heart
Joyful	Spleen, Kidney, Liver, Heart, Circulation-Sex
Kind	Spleen, Heart, Liver, Lungs
Liked	Spleen, Heart, Liver, Circulation-Sex
Loved	Spleen, Heart, Liver, Circulation-Sex
Loving	Spleen, Heart, Liver, Circulation-Sex
Normal	All of them
Optimistic	Spleen, Heart, Kidney, Bladder, Liver

Popular	Spleen, Heart, Liver, Circulation Sex, Lungs
Quiet	Lungs, Kidney
Real	Spleen, Heart, Circulation-Sex, Lungs, Liver
Relaxed	Triple Warmer, Stomach
Right	Large Intestine, Stomach, Liver
Safe	Triple Warmer
Satisfied	Stomach, Lungs, Circulation-Sex, Liver
Strong	Liver, Kidney, Heart, Spleen
Successful	All of them, but especially: Spleen, Liver, Kidney
Unusual	All of them, but especially: Liver
Upbeat	Spleen, Heart, Bladder

Negative Attributes and Emotions

*If you DID CIRCLE any of the following words
in Exercise 1, it could be an indication that:*

- *The energy flowing through the related meridian is weak,
unbalanced or blocked.*
- *You might be feeling overwhelmed by the following negative
feelings and emotions:*

Attribute	Related meridian(s)
Angry	Liver, Gallbladder, Heart
Blocked	Liver, Gallbladder, Large Intestine
Competitive	Heart, Gallbladder
Confused	Circulation-Sex, Small Intestine, Stomach
Controlling	Gallbladder, Small Intestine, Large Intestine

Cynical	Bladder, Lungs, Heart
Disappointed	Heart, Circulation-Sex
Empty	Bladder, Kidney, Large Intestine, Lungs
Exhausted	Triple Warmer, Spleen
Failure	Liver, Heart, Bladder, Kidney, Stomach
Fearful	Bladder, Kidney
Frustrated	Liver, Gallbladder, Circulation-Sex, Large Intestine
Guilty	Liver, Heart
Jealous	Liver, Stomach, Gallbladder
Judged	Liver, Heart
Judgmental	Liver, Gallbladder
Loud	Circulation-Sex, Gallbladder, Small Intestine
Numb	Kidney, Heart, Lungs
Outsider	Lungs, Liver, Heart
Overwhelmed	Triple Warmer
Phony	Liver, Kidney, Spleen
Quiet	Lungs, Circulation-Sex
Reserved	Lungs, Circulation-Sex, Liver
Rigid	Large Intestine, Liver, Gallbladder
Selfish	Spleen, Heart, Small Intestine
Shy	Kidney, Lungs
Stressed	Triple Warmer
Stuck	Kidney, Bladder, Small Intestine, Heart, Large Intestine
Switched-off	Lungs, Spleen, Heart
Tired	Spleen, Triple Warmer
Unfriendly	Spleen, Gallbladder, Lungs

Unpopular	Triple Warmer
Unusual	All of them, especially Liver
Upset	Gallbladder, Liver, Circulation-Sex
Vengeful	Gallbladder, Large Intestine
Worried	Stomach, Bladder, Small Intestine
Wrong	Liver, Bladder

The first way to start joining the dots

Identify which meridians keep coming up as being weak, blocked or unbalanced in some way, and make a note of them. Next, take a look at the *Quick Reference Tool: Meridians and Their Associated Physical Issues* on pg. 181, and see which physical issues are linked to any of the meridians you've written down.

If something starts to ring a bell for you, head over to the Appendixes in the back of the book, and experiment with some of the different tools you'll find there to get your energy and emotions balanced and flowing again.

The second way to start joining the dots

The following exercise can help you to identify your main physical issues, which you can then use to work backwards to identify any blocked emotions, using the *Quick Reference Tables* on pages 179 and 182.

EXERCISE 2: Identify your physical issues and / or chronic illnesses

Take a few moments and try to answer the following questions:

- **What illnesses have you had, in the last 12 months?** (Note: Include even the 'small stuff,' like colds, coughs, piles and headaches.)

- **Are any of these illnesses recurrent?** (i.e., you get them repeatedly)

- **Are any of these illnesses chronic?** (i.e., they have periods where they flare up, and periods where they calm down, but you're never fully free of them)

- **What physical problems do you have?** (aches and pains, broken bones, pigeon toes, poor eyesight, etc.)

- **Do you have any autoimmune diseases?** (more common autoimmune diseases include things like eczema, asthma, allergies, fibromyalgia, MS, etc.)

Hopefully, you don't have loads of things on your list. If you do, try to prioritize them by putting a number '1' next to the illness or physical issue that's the most serious, or is having the biggest negative impact on your quality of life.

That's your priority.

(If you have multiple physical issues, try to rank them according to severity. If that's overwhelming, just stick with Number One on your list for now, and revisit this exercise periodically to see what your next priority should be.)

Now that you know what your physical issues are, check to see what meridian, or meridians, they could be associated with, using the 'Meridians and Their Associated Physical Issues' tool below.

Simply look up your physical issue, and make a note of the meridian it's often connected to. Start to look for patterns, or a recurring theme, then answer the following question:

Q: What meridian, or meridians, seems to be coming up the most often?

MERIDIANS AND THEIR ASSOCIATED PHYSICAL ISSUES

QUICK REFERENCE TABLE 1

Stomach

Acid indigestion; reflux

Allergies

Bags under the eyes

Bloating and gas

Digestion issues

Hunger

Lip and mouth sores

Neck pain

Nervous Tension

Ovary issues

Sinusitis

Sore throat

Stomach aches

Stomach ulcers

Tender Breasts

Weight Problems

Spleen

Allergies

Anemia

Anything to do with blood

Carpal Tunnel Syndrome

Cysts

Diabetes

Edema (swelling)

Fertility / pregnancy issues

Hypoglycemia

Immunodeficiency issues

Infections

Lymph nodes

Varicose veins

Weakness (general feelings of)

Weight Issues

Heart

Angina

Arteries

Bleeding gums

Blood pressure (high or low)

Chest pains

Circulation issues

Dizziness

Eczema

Heart issues

Sleep issues

Swollen glands

Small Intestine

Abdominal issues or pain

Beer bellies

Knee pain

Shoulder pain

Tinnitus / ear problems

Weakness in legs

Bladder

Ankle pain / weakness

Arthritis

Baldness

Back pain (general)

Calf pain

Elbow issues

Fallen arches / flat feet

Headaches (at the front of the head)

Joint pain

Nervous system issues

Osteoporosis

Sciatica

Scoliosis

Kidney

Acne

Bone weakness / issues

Back pain (lower back)

Ear issues; earaches

Edema

Eyesight

Infertility / impotence

Low libido

Prostrate

Swollen ankles

Tooth / gum issues

Circulation-Sex

Hormones

Impotence

Prostrate issues

Sacrum issues

Sexual issues

Sore breasts, nipples, or buttocks

Triple Warmer

Adrenal exhaustion or burn-out

Allergies

Asthma

Diabetes

Fever

Hives

Hormonal issues

Hypoglycemia

Menopause

Mood swings

PMS

Temperate issues (too hot; too cold)

Weight issues

Liver

Blurry vision

Candida

Eye infections / diseases

Fungal diseases

Hepatitis

Hypertension

Jaundice

Low sperm count

Menopause

PMS

Toenail problems (thick; yellow)

Toxicity

Gallbladder

Arthritis

Bitter taste in the mouth

Blood pressure (high)

Gallstones

Hip pain or issues

Jaw pain; TMJ

Leg pain (side of the legs)

Migraine headaches

'One-sided' issues, including headaches

Shingles

Teeth grinding

Lung

Bronchitis

Chest infections

Colds

Coughs

Flu

Pleurisy

Pneumonia

Respiratory issues

Shortness of breath

Skin issues

Tuberculosis

Large Intestine

Colic pain

Colonic issues

Constipation; Haemorrhoids

Diarrhoea

Herpes

Hip problems

Mineral deficiency

Nose issues

Toothache

When you work with Energy Medicine and meridians, you'll often find that many of your physical symptoms and issues are connected to the same blockage in a particular emotion, and its related meridian. When you work on what's really underlying your main physical issue, it often happens that a lot of your more minor problems will disappear on their own, as a result.

EXERCISE 3: The Shortcut

If going through lists and circling stuff is just not your style, or if you already know you have a physical issue and just want a quick reference tool to show you what negative emotions may be underneath the problem, you'll find just the ticket below.

If you've got acid indigestion, say, it'll take just two seconds to reference 'Stomach' in the following Table and see what's probably causing the problem at the emotional level: worry, anxiety and day-to-day stress.

Bingo! Now you know what you need to work on, and it took you a whole two seconds to figure it out.

QUICK REFERENCE TABLE 1	
Meridian	**Associated Negative Emotion**
Stomach	Anxiety, pessimism, worry, stress, stinginess
Spleen	People pleasing, 'suffering martyr,' unable to assimilate knowledge and ideas
Heart	Heartache, broken-heartedness, sadness, jealousy
Small Intestine	Confusion, indecision, 'divided'
Bladder	Scared, fearful of the outside world, despair, cynicism
Kidney	Loneliness, toxic shame, traumatized, 'frozen'
Circulation-Sex	Frustration, over-commitment, disconnected from self
Triple Warmer	Fight / flight / freeze, overwhelmed, primal fear
Gallbladder	Anger (at others), harsh judgment, criticism
Liver	Beating myself up, guilt, can't accept or like the self, toxic shame, anger at the self
Lung	Profound sadness, grief, yearning, detachment from others, massive disappointment
Large Intestine	Control-freak, can't let go, can't surrender to God/others

Remember that you're particularly interested in trying to spot a *repressed* emotion that may now be showing up as a physical issue. Emotions get repressed when you don't accept them, validate them or let yourself connect to them consciously, so pay particular attention to any emotion listed for your particular meridian where you:

■ Experience a strong reaction to the thought that you may have it (such as indignation, outrage, upset, shock, denial or fear).

■ Think or know you may have had that problem in the past, but now you believe it's gone.

If either of these things apply (and especially if both of these things apply) you've probably just come a huge step closer to identifying the mystery emotion that's causing so much havoc in your life.

Unless you are 100% sure that you:

1. Got the Divinely-tailored message that particular emotion was coming to teach you about what you needed to change or fix in your life and

2. Acted on it – then that negative emotion didn't just disappear; it went underground.

This can happen even if you've been trying to work through your emotions in therapy for years.

If you have a problem or issue that isn't specifically covered here, simply take it back to God, ask Him to point you in the right direction.

Tell me again: Once I know what the real problem is, how do I fix it?

Your bit of the equation boils down to this:

- Get God involved in the process

- Work out which bits need fixing (Anger? Compassion? Worry? Lack of love?)

- Apply an appropriate Energy Medicine tool or technique to the related meridian

- Let God do His thing.

In Appendix 3 at the back, you'll find some real-life Client Case Files, illustrating more ways of applying the 'Talk to God and Fix Your Health' system to identifying and resolving physical and emotional issues.

I know this method can sound like the long-haul. Why should you bother doing all this 'emotional' stuff, when you can just pop the pill and have it over and done with? I'm going to try and answer that question in the next chapter. Hang on.

RECAP

- Negative emotions and bad characteristics can block the Divine energy flowing through your body, and cause you a number of emotional and physical problems.

- And also vice versa! 'Blocked' energy in your body can cause you to develop negative emotions, bad characteristics, and physical issues.

- You can start to diagnose the 'block' in your Divine energy by looking at your physical and / or emotional symptoms, and working backwards.

- Blocks can be dissolved with prayer, and by simply becoming aware of what the real root of the problem is, along with a wide range of Energy Medicine and energy psychology techniques - many of which you can do safely and easily at home.

Chapter 9

Why Conventional Medicine Can't Always Fix The Real Problem

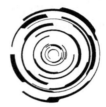

A man sits down to eat his meal. Unbeknownst to him, the food he's about to eat contains a deadly poison. He doesn't know that, but we do. What's the best way to approach the problem? Do we run over to him, and warn him not to eat the food? Or do we wait until he eats it and starts to feel really ill, and then give him the magic potion that may save his life?

In the above analogy, the correct approach seems like a no-brainer: *of course* we're going to run over to him, and warn him not to eat the poisonous food! The advantages of this approach is that it's much easier, faster and less complicated, and it's for sure going to save his life.

So why go down the other route? Let's make the analogy even sharper, by saying that the man with the magic potion wants a thousand gold coins for it (which the patient may or may not have), and that the magic potion itself isn't 100% guaranteed to work, and that even if it does work, it could cause the patient some very unpleasant and potentially life-threatening side effects.

Given all of this, who in their right mind would pick the 'magic potion' option?

Yet what we've just described is the basic difference between God-based holistic health techniques, in all its different forms, and conventional Western medicine. We *know* that people get sick from eating unhealthy, artificially flavored foods that are high in sugar, chemicals and other poisonous substances. We *know* that people who spend all day sitting passively in front of a screen are gearing themselves up for health problems down the road, if they don't take steps to exercise properly and look after their bodies. We *know* that negative emotions like jealousy, anger, sadness and hatred cause all sorts of mental and physical issues.

But how many Western doctors ever try to encourage their patients to stop doing all the stuff that's making them sick? In fairness to the physicians, a lot of us don't want to listen. To return to our analogy, it's like someone running over to tell the man he's about to eat deadly poison, and the man simply ignores him and carries on.

But what if three people ran up to tell him the same thing? Or 15 people? Or 100? At some point, even the most stubborn mule-head would hopefully have to get the message, and put down his fork.

But that's not what's happening. Instead, for every one person out there who's popping up to tell us about the dangers of our negative lifestyle choices, there's at least another six, or sixty, or six hundred, popping up to discount it all and wave their magic potions in our faces.

"OK, the food *may* be poisonous. But so what? It's delicious! And after you've enjoyed your meal to the max, all you have to do is take our magic potion, and hey presto, we just took care of the consequences…"

Taking responsibility for your own health

What it all boils down to is that you are responsible for you own health, and for the healthy functioning of your body and soul. If a person already ate the poison, unwittingly or not, then Western medicine's 'magic potions' are probably the most sensible option to pick, at least in the short-term.

But there is another, better way out there, and as soon as you make even the smallest effort to connect your health to God, you'll start to see that healing is abundantly available to you, in any number of gentle, cheap and effective ways.

Modern medicine is big business - more than a trillion dollars a year, by some estimates. Everyone has to take responsibility for themselves, and to ascertain to the best of their ability if the information they're being told is primarily focused on getting them well ('don't eat the poison!') or paying someone else's mortgage ('buy my magic potion!').

Iatrogenic Illnesses - Kill or Cure?

I only learned the term 'iatrogenic illness' when I started researching the facts on how many people are actually being unnecessarily hurt or even killed by Western medicine.

'Iatrogenic' means illness or death that occurs as a result of the treatment itself, which is occurring in much greater numbers than anyone is talking about. Part of the problem is that there are so many vested interests in keeping the multi-trillion dollar model of modern medicine going exactly as it is, that it's very difficult to get a clear picture of what is actually happening at the human level of doctors and their patients.

Even when honest mistakes are being made - and how can they not be? - it's simply not part of modern medical culture to own up to them. Making mistakes makes you a 'bad' doctor... making mistakes can get you sued... making mistakes is something that doctors simply don't do...

That's why there are no reported errors in medical procedures, and precious little follow-up. The assumption seems to be that if you get better, it's because of the amazing drugs, surgery and care you received; and if you get worse or die, that's your own fault.

But the research is starting to come through - in dribs and drabs - to prove that modern medicine is not the panacea it pretends to be. One of the most well-researched and credible reports comes from The Nutrition Institute of America, and you can read that report's main findings below.

Probably the report's most shocking claim is that the American medical system is the leading cause of death and injury in the U.S. - even edging out death due to heart disease or cancer.

If this sounds incredible, just take a moment and think about the people you know, in your own life, who were let down by modern medicine and then multiply that by six billion people.

Clearly, for all its highly publicized success stories, the invasive 'drugs and surgery' approach that epitomizes Western medicine comes with a number of major drawbacks and risks.

Many of us acknowledge that, but what's the alternative? When your kid is running a high temperature, or you've got stabbing pains in your chest, what else are you supposed to do?

It's a good question, and not a simple or easy one to answer. Even with all its drawbacks, Western medicine is probably still always the best choice for acute, life-threatening emergencies. But hopefully it's becoming clearer that given all the risks entailed in methods for a 'cure,' going back to basics and putting the focus on prevention, and putting God center stage in the healing picture, has to be the better way to go.

Headline facts from 'Death by Medicine'

- This fully referenced report shows the number of people having in-hospital, adverse reactions to prescribed drugs to be 2.2 million per year.

- The number of unnecessary antibiotics prescribed annually for viral infections is 20 million per year.

- The number of unnecessary medical and surgical procedures performed annually is 7.5 million per year.

- The number of people exposed to unnecessary hospitalization annually is 8.9 million per year.

- The most stunning statistic, however, is that the total number of deaths caused by conventional medicine is an astounding 783,936 per year. It is now evident that the American medical system is the leading cause of death and injury in the U.S. (By contrast, the number of deaths attributable to heart disease in 2001 was 699,697, while the number of deaths attributable to cancer was 553,251.)

- The estimated 10-year total of 7.8 million iatrogenic deaths is more than all the casualties from all the wars fought by the U.S. throughout its entire history.

The Spiritual View

Top spiritual guide Shalom Arush explains the dilemma of using Western medicine to cure your health issues very clearly:

"Illness is like a warning light and siren, presaging man to change his ways before he can reclaim his health. Medicine, in contrast, is a Band-Aid on an open wound, a flimsy patch that suppresses the body's natural reactions. In fact, medicines may be even more hazardous to one's health than the illness itself...medicine is like a bandage that covers, but doesn't truly heal."

That's the spiritual view, but Andrew Weil, MD, said something very similar in his book "Spontaneous Healing," and emphasized that he was particularly uneasy that the suppressive nature of much of modern medicine is just storing up larger health problems for patients in the future.

The medical statistics quoted above appear to be showing this very clearly, and it bears repeating: according to at least one credible, well-researched report, conventional medicine is the biggest cause of death in the USA, ahead of cancer, heart disease and all of the other big nasties.

Why talk to God about your health?

Now that we've looked at some of the limitations of conventional medicine, let's just take a brief look at why the 'Talk to God and Fix Your Health' approach is better. Why is the approach set out in this book any more useful, effective or reliable than anything else out there?

Firstly, the focus of this book is firmly on 'prevention' instead of a 'cure.' It's about helping you, the reader, to identify the negative attitudes, emotions and lifestyle choices that are actually making you sick, before you even get anywhere near actually needing to visit a doctor.

Your body is just the wrapping paper for your soul. God is really all there is, and God's energy is what is animating you, everyone and everything around you. That's exactly what Einstein told us, more than 100 years ago, when he came up with his famous formula: e=mc2.

'Energy Is All There Is' - Albert Einstein

Atoms are the building blocks of our physical reality, but every atom is one part nucleus to between 10,000 and 100,000 parts empty space.

Everything you regard as being 'solid matter' is actually mostly empty space that's held together by a cloud of particles that are effectively composed of light.

Mind-bending as it sounds, even in the strictly 'physical' realm of Quantum Physics, human beings are composed of light and space. This has enormous implications for your physical health. To quote clinical psychologist David Feinstein, writing in the book 'Energy Medicine for Women':

"The paradigm of worldview embraced by Western medicine is a century behind the paradigm used by modern physics."

What Einstein first told us more than a century ago, and what Quantum Physics is proving in more amazing detail all the time, is that physical matter is made up of energy. That's true for inanimate objects like the chair you sit on, the bed you lie on and the car you drive. And it's certainly true for living matter like you and your physical body.

Energy, i.e., God, is all there is.

Choose health

Every second, you can make a choice that's going to bring you closer to God, good energy and good health, or the opposite.

The food you eat affects your health. The way you act towards yourself and others affects your health. Your positive and negative beliefs affect your health. Your thoughts, emotions, words and deeds - it all affects your health. Once you know that everything you do, every single second of your life, is affecting your health for good or for bad, it's very empowering.

It means that you no longer need to waste time, money and effort tracking down 'experts' or 'gurus' to tell you what's wrong, and how to fix it. With the basic tools and guidance contained in this book, you can start to piece the clues together for yourself.

What's the message?

When you start to use the 'Talk to God' approach, staying healthy no longer depends on you only eating salad, regularly taking your meds, or getting everything 'diagnosed' within a split second of discovering it. It takes so much of the pressure off, because this approach opens up a whole other spiritual dimension to your health and healing, enabling you to find so many more ways you can be cured. Instead of having a panic attack about every little ache or pain, your focus will shift more to working out what message God is trying to give you.

God wants you to change. He wants you to improve. If He, in His wisdom, makes you ill, He wants you to think about WHY He's doing that, and not just to pull in all your connections to get an appointment with 'the top guy' at the hospital.

I know, I know: this is hard-core, isn't it? That's why so many people prefer the pills and 'magic potions' approach. But that doesn't change the reality, that: *The single best preventative measure for staying healthy, physically and spiritually, is to develop a strong relationship with God, where you talk to Him every day, and where you try to decipher the hints He's sending you about what to work on, before they manifest as harsh illnesses or physical problems.*

However big the problem, however serious the disease, however bad the diagnosis, it's never too late to apply the 'Talk to God and Fix Your Health' approach set out in this book. God is the single best cure I know of, and He works for everything.

You can still use doctors if you want to

Now, there's a big clarification I need to make at this stage, so please pay attention: I'm not saying don't go to doctors. What I *am* saying, is don't decide anything before you talk to God about it. You can combine talking to God with any other healthcare model that appeals to you: surgery, medication, juice fasts, homeopathy, cranio-sacral therapy, Chinese medicine, naturopathy, aromatherapy, zoo therapy - the options are endless.

As long as you're connecting it all back to God, somehow, you'll get there in the end. And if you're not? Remember what we said at the beginning of the book: either the medicine, surgery or therapy won't work, or it won't work very well, or it won't work for long, or the original problem will disappear, but a new one will pop up instead.

Why? Because you got stuck trying to deal with the symptoms, instead of working on the root. But when you talk to God to fix your health, you'll get to the heart of the problem, fast, and fix your health at every level.

The importance of free choice

So many of us have been raised with the notion that we have to outsource decisions about the most important areas in our life to 'experts' of all stripes, that it sounds almost irresponsible for us to try to think for ourselves. But the 'experts' don't have to live with the consequences of their advice: you do. The 'experts' aren't the ones who pay the price when their advice turns out to be wrong or seriously flawed: you do.

But perhaps the most telling reason why you should take back the responsibility for your life and health from the 'experts' is because you are the person who is best placed to make these decisions. Who really knows you, the way you do? Who can feel your feelings, or your symptoms, the way you can? Who can understand your aspirations, or dream your dreams? Only you!

Occasionally, you may still need the advice of a God-fearing medical 'expert,' or an authentic spiritual guide, to get you moving in the right direction again when you get stuck. That's fine - as long as you still retain your free choice, and you understand that the person with the most knowledge about you, and the best advice to help you, is ultimately you. The truly wise people know this already, which is why they will never try to scare you, manipulate you or bully you into doing what they say.

What they will do, is gently guide you and encourage you to educate yourself about what is really going on in your life, and to take everything back to God, before making any firm decisions. That Divine part of us called our soul already contains all the advice, help and information we need to be the people God created us to be.

So trust yourself! Believe yourself! If you're regularly in touch with God, He will give you all the ideas, insights and tools you need to get, and stay, truly healthy.

RECAP

- Western medicine puts the emphasis firmly on 'cure'; talking to God puts the emphasis on preventing ill-health in the first place.

- Taking medication, even over-the-counter medication taken as pre-scribed, is not risk-free, and can cause a number of side effects and illnesses, ranging from very mild to life-threatening.

- The Talk to God approach encourages you to take responsibility for your own healthcare and well-being back from the medical professionals. You know far more about the real, root causes of your mental and physical problems.

- You can combine Talking to God with any other healthcare approach you care to mention.

Chapter 10

Easy Ways To Stay Healthy

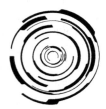

In this final chapter, I want to share some concluding tips with you about staying healthy.

Now, when I say 'staying healthy' that doesn't mean that you'll never get a cold again, or another headache, or a sore throat. Following this prescription doesn't mean that you'll ALWAYS be 100% healthy, 100% of the time. There are a few reasons why I can't make that guarantee:

Firstly, **I'm not God.**

Sometimes things can get so out of kilter in your life that only a bout of serious, or chronic illness can shake you out of habits and destructive patterns that, otherwise, you'd find it far too hard to break out of by yourself. God knows that, and that's often why He's sending you the 'big, nasty stuff,' to help you to make big shifts in your life and in your outlook that would otherwise be impossible to achieve.

We've all heard of people who had near-death experiences, or recovered from a bout of something apparently 'terminal,' who went on to make wholesale changes in their lives. Overnight, many of them became much more caring, compassionate, humble and genuine human beings, determined to build the world in whatever way they could, with the extra time they'd been given.

Another reason why you might follow this prescription and still get seriously ill is because (I'm sorry to break this to you...) you're not meant to be down here on the planet forever. Sometimes, it's just time for your soul to go back to God, and serious illness is often the route by which that occurs.

The Fourth Reason Why You Get Sick

Lastly, even the wisest and most saintly human being on the planet can't always understand God's ways. If we could, we'd be God.

99% of the time, illness is just a message, and the approach set out in this book will work like clockwork to help you work out what's happening, why, and how you need to respond. The other 1% of the time, it won't work like that at all. Why not? Because God is not always predictable, and His system of spiritual accounting is completely beyond human comprehension.

Sometimes, God decrees that a person needs to get sick, and there's nothing that person needs to fix, work on or change. The good news is, that usually only happens to the holiest of saintly people (so unless that's an accurate description of you, don't worry about it too much).

Otherwise, if you're living the life God intended for you, picking up the clues He's sending you via your health when they're still at the 'small' stage; AND it's not yet your time to go - then the Talk to God and Fix Your Health formula I've set out in this book will help to keep you in tip-top shape, spiritually, emotionally and physically.

God loves you

If there's one idea I'd like you to take away from this book, it's this: God loves you.

Not only that, He loves you 100%. Not only that, He loves you unconditionally, and He really wants to help you feel good again. I know that can be hard to believe when you're struggling with health issues, but when you make even the smallest possible move towards including God in your health and well-being, you will reap enormous rewards from it. You don't have to follow the ideas and the concepts in this book slavishly to achieve massive and permanent improvements in your state of mind and your physical health: you just need to be willing to get God involved.

Remember, the stronger your daily connection to God, the healthier your soul will be, the healthier your emotional state, and the healthier your physical body will get. And it's never too early - or too late - to start. Whatever your age, whatever your current state of physical health, however strong - or weak - your relationship with God currently is, even the smallest effort you make to get God more involved in your health and well-being will pay out massive dividends for you, in every area of your life.

When you're spiritually healthy, the rest of your life starts to fall into place much easier, and even when you do get your periodic difficulties and challenges, you'll come through them much faster and easier, and they'll ultimately only strengthen you.

So without any further ado, let me share with you the 'Talk to God Ten Commandments' for fixing your health:

The Talk to God Ten Commandments for Fixing Your Health

1. Talk to God every single day - even if it's only for a minute.

2. Try to look for the real, spiritual root of your physical problems, before popping the Tylenol (or at least, at the same time as popping the Tylenol).

3. Keep your internal and external environment as 'clean' as you can - minimize junk food, junk habits and junk conversations.

4. Stay away from negative people, as much as you possibly can.

5. Love yourself! Even if you're still making a big mess of things, God loves every tiny effort you make to build the world, and to improve, and to bring Him into your life.

6. Don't beat yourself up for having negative emotions - they're just the tools God is using to help you heal, spiritually and physically. Accept them, work out the message, and then let them go.

7. Don't panic when you get sick, even if the conventional diagnosis is bad. If you include God in your health, everything can turn around for the best, even miraculously.

8. Take back responsibility for your health from the experts - you know far more about what's causing your problems than they do.

9. Remember that every day is a present. Use it to put more love, compassion, kindness and joy into your life, your relationships, and your surroundings.

10. Pay attention to the small stuff - if you get the message at that level, then God doesn't need to ramp things up to get your attention.

The last word is to remind you that you are so much more than your body. The 'real' you is your soul, and it's only beautiful and good. The more you strengthen your connection to God, the more that real, holy, beautiful you will shine through.

Appendix 1

Basic Guide to Balancing Your Meridians

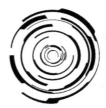

General information

For the purposes of this book, there are four main ways that you can easily and safely balance the energy in your meridians by yourself, in the comfort of your own home. They include:

- Tracing the meridians

- Massaging the relevant neurolymphatic points for around 10 seconds (on the chest and back)

- Strengthening and sedating the acupressure points

- Holding the relevant neurovascular points on the head

1. How to Trace Your Meridians

Each meridian has its own pathway, and directional flow, in the body.

To trace a meridian, simply use the flat of your hand to 'trace' the pathway (as shown in the pictures below) from the start to the finish. Your hand can be touching your body, or held 2-3 centimeters away from it. Don't worry about doing it too precisely; if you're using the flat of your palm, you're covering a wide enough area to be sure of being in the right place.

Ideally, aim to trace your meridians every day, in the order given below:

Fig. 11.1 - Central

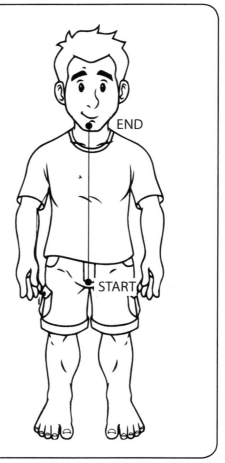

TO TRACE CENTRAL MERIDIAN:

1. Begin at your pubic bone.

2. Using both hands, trace straight up the middle of your body, to your lower lip.

Night / Midnight

Fig. 11.2 - Governing

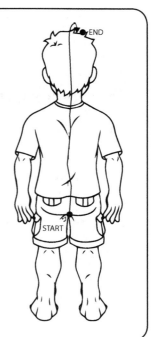

TO TRACE GOVERNING MERIDIAN:

1. Using both hands, begin at your sacrum (the bony knob at the very bottom of your spine) and bring both hands up the center of your back, as far as they'll go.

2. When you get to your shoulder blades, leave the first hand on your back, then take the second hand over your head and shoulders, and try to get your hands to touch (if they can't, imagine them touching).

3. Take the second hand up over the back of your head, over your forehead, to the top lip.

Day / Noon

Fig. 11.3 - Stomach

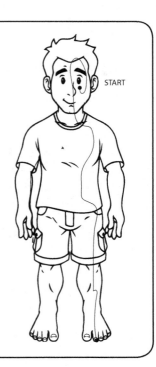

TO TRACE STOMACH MERIDIAN:

1. Using both hands, place your fingertips on your cheekbones, below your eyes. Circle around the outside of your eyes, over your eyebrows, and straight down your nose and chin.

2. Trace out across your clavicles, down over your nipples, then down the center of your stomach.

3. Flare out again at the hips, then continue tracing down the front of your leg, to your second toe.

7-9 AM

Fig. 11.4 - Spleen

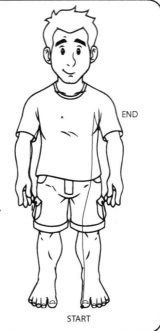

TO TRACE SPLEEN MERIDIAN:

1. Start at the outside tip of your big toe.

2. Trace straight up the inside of your leg, straight up over the stomach and rib cage, to your armpits.

3. Trace back down to the bottom of your rib cage. Repeat on the other side.

9-11 AM

Fig. 11-5 - Heart

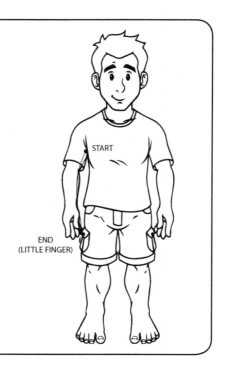

TO TRACE HEART MERIDIAN:

1. To begin, put your hand under your armpit.

2. Trace along the bottom of your arm, to the pinkie finger. Make sure you really pull the energy off the pinkie finger. Repeat on the other side.

11 AM-1 PM

NOTE: NEVER TRACE THE HEART MERIDIAN BACKWARDS

Fig. 11.6 - Small Intestine

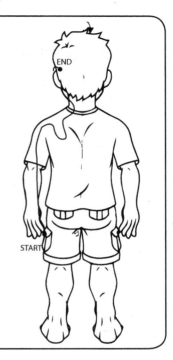

TO TRACE SMALL INTESTINE MERIDIAN:

1. Start at the tip of your little finger. Trace up the outside of your arm.

2. Trace across the back of your shoulder, and drop down around your shoulder blade.

3. Trace up the back of your neck, then come around your neck to the front of your face.

4. Trace to your cheekbone, then take it back to just by your ear. Repeat on the other side.

1–3 PM

Fig. 11.7 - Bladder

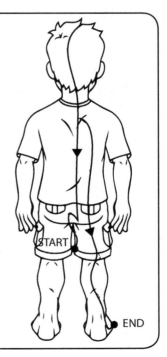

TO TRACE BLADDER MERIDIAN:

1. Begin at the top upper lip, and bring both hands over the crown of your head, and down your spine, to the top of your buttocks.

2. Pause, then indent your hands and trace around the bottom of your buttocks.

3. Take both hands up to the top of your back (thumbs by armpits), and trace straight down the backs of the legs, and off the little toe.

3–5 PM

Fig. 11.8 - Kidney

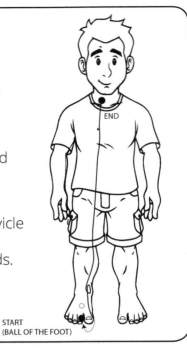

TO TRACE KIDNEY MERIDIAN:

1. To begin, use both hands, and press in on the ball of each foot (do both feet together).

2. Trace up to the ankle, and circle around the ankle bone.

3. Trace straight up the inside of the leg, over the rib cage, to just below the clavicle bones (the K-27 points). Vigorously massage these points for a few seconds.

5–7 PM

END

START
(BALL OF THE FOOT)

Fig. 11.9 - Circulation-Sex

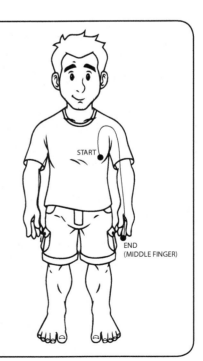

TO TRACE CIRCULATION-SEX MERIDIAN:

1. Place your hand over your nipple.

2. Trace along your inner arm, until the tip of your third (middle) finger.

3. Repeat on the other side.

7–9 PM

START

END
(MIDDLE FINGER)

Fig. 11.10 - Triple Warmer

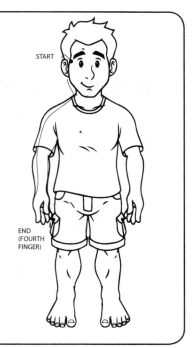

TO TRACE TRIPLE WARMER MERIDIAN:

1. Using both hands, place your fingertips at your temples, then trace around the back of your ears, and down the back of your neck to your shoulders.

2. Continue tracing down the outside of your arm, ending at the fourth (ring) finger.

3. Repeat on the other side.

9–11 PM

Fig. 11.11 - Gallbladder

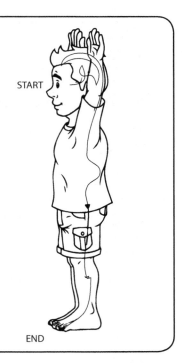

TO TRACE GALLBLADDER MERIDIAN:

1. Using both hands, begin at the corner of your eyebrows; make a circle on your temples, then trace back to behind the ears.

2. Bring both hands together to your forehead, then back across the crown of your head, and down the back of your neck.

3. Trace down the sides of your body, going back on the ribcage, then forward again on the hips, down the sides of your legs, then off your fourth toe.

11 PM–1 AM

Fig. 11.12 - Liver

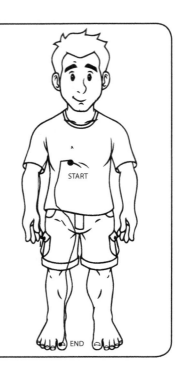

TO TRACE LIVER MERIDIAN:

1. Start at the inside of your big toe.

2. Trace straight up the inside of your legs, flaring out at the hips.

3. Trace up over your stomach, then horizontally under your pecs, stopping in line with your nipples. Repeat on the other side.

1–3 AM

Fig. 11.13 - Lung

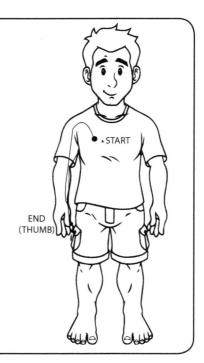

TO TRACE LUNG MERIDIAN:

1. Place your hand on your chest, over your lung.

2. Trace straight down the inside of your arm, to your thumb. Make sure to pull the energy off your thumb.

3. Repeat on the other side.

3–5 AM

Fig. 11.14 - Large Intestine

TO TRACE LARGE INTESTINE MERIDIAN:

1. Start at the tip of your pointer finger. Trace up the outside of your arm, and around your shoulder.

2. Continue tracing across your clavicle bones to your throat.

3. Trace up over the bottom of your face (to the side of your chin) to the tip of your nose, then trace back to the 'flare' of your nostril. Repeat on the other side.

5–7 AM

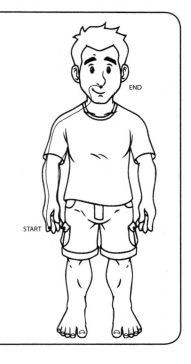

2. How to Massage Your Neurolymphatic Points

Using the diagram below, identify which neurolymphatic points are associated with the particular meridian you need to work on, and simply massage the relevant points for around 10 seconds. If energy is blocked there, it will probably feel tender and a bit sore. Once the stagnant energy has been broken up and 'moved on,' the tenderness will reduce, and even disappear.

Fig. 11.15

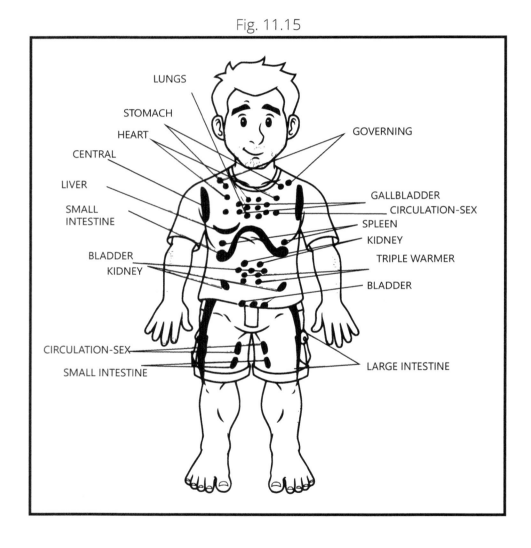

3. How to Strengthen and Sedate Your Acupressure Points

General guidelines

If you think a lot of your meridians are unbalanced, OR you're pretty sure that your Triple Warmer Meridian is over-reactive and switched on most of the time, (leading to feelings of overwhelm, and regular fight /flight / freeze impulses) then use the acupressure points for sedating the Triple Warmer Meridian before working with the other meridians.

An over-reactive Triple Warmer 'steals' the energy from the other meridians, leaving them weak and / or blocked. When you sedate your Triple Warmer, the first thing it does is shoot some of that stolen energy back to the other meridians it came from, giving you some energetic 'juice' to work with.

How to hold your acupressure strengthening and sedating points

The procedure is the same for sedating or strengthening:

1. Gently but firmly hold the first set of points (marked 'first') for between 2-3 minutes, or until you can feel a pulse. Then, hold these 'first' points on the other side of the body for the same amount of time.

2. Then, hold the second set of points (marked 'second') for between 1 and 2 minutes, or until you can feel a pulse. Switch sides and repeat.

Do this once a day, or three times a day, as the need arises.

"When should I 'sedate' and when should I 'strengthen'?"

You can safely experiment with these techniques to see what works for you, because acupressure is non-invasive, and even if you don't actually need a particular procedure, it won't do you any harm. (That said, I'm still including some safety data info below, just to be on the safe side.) But the general guidelines are as follows:

SEDATE: When you are dealing with tension, pain or a blockage on a particular meridian. Pain is usually a sign of excess energy being present in the meridian.

STRENGTHEN: When you're dealing with chronically weak energy in a particular meridian.

Are there any safety issues?

As mentioned, acupressure is non-invasive, and shouldn't do you any harm, even if you don't actually need a particular procedure. That said, there are a few provisos you should take into account:

Always strengthen Heart and Spleen Meridians

You won't even find the points for sedating the Heart Meridian here, because it's not a good idea to sedate the heart unless you're an acupressure guru of many years standing (and even then, maybe still not...). In a similar vein, you should NEVER trace the Heart Meridian backwards. Also, because Spleen energy is chronically weak in nearly everyone today, it's nearly always a good idea to just strengthen Spleen.

An exception could be if you're experiencing blood clots, or something similar. In those circumstances, sedate Spleen first, but then strengthen it again immediately afterwards.

Guidelines for pregnant women

You should avoid using any acupressure techniques on the abdominal area during pregnancy, and you should also work more gently than otherwise.

People with life-threatening illnesses

Consult with your physicians before doing acupressure.

People with serious burns / recent scars

Don't press directly on these areas until they've healed, which usually takes at least a month.

Use your common sense

Common sense and intuition are the key to getting acupressure to work for you. If something doesn't feel right, or is causing you a lot of discomfort and pain - stop.

Ask God what's going on, and then try a different approach to solving the problem.

The Acupressure Strengthening And Sedating Points

Fig. 11.16 - Stomach Strengthening

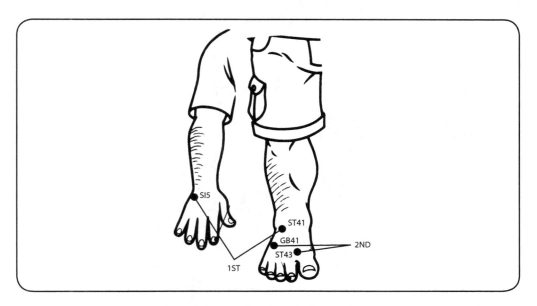

Fig. 11.17 - Stomach Sedating

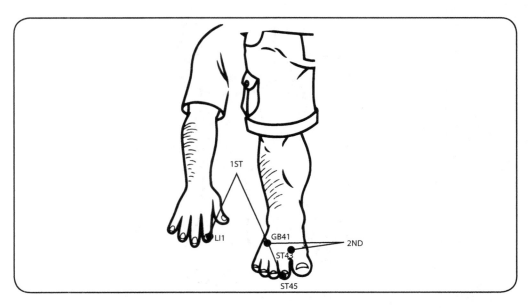

Fig. 11.18 - Spleen Strengthening

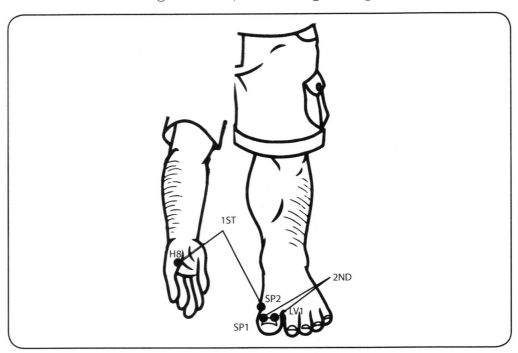

Fig. 11.19 - Spleen Sedating

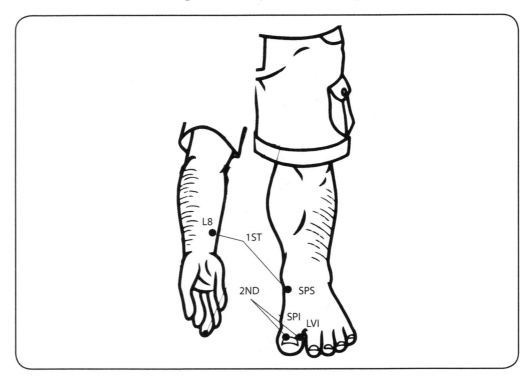

Fig. 11.20 - Heart Strengthening

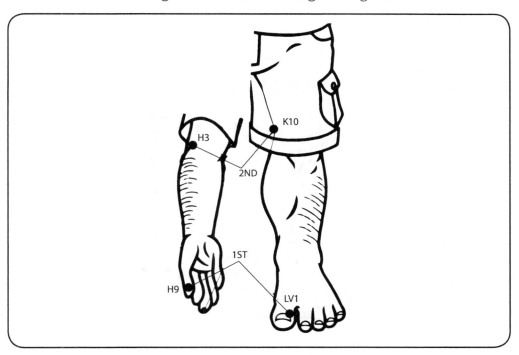

Fig. 11.21 - Heart Sedating

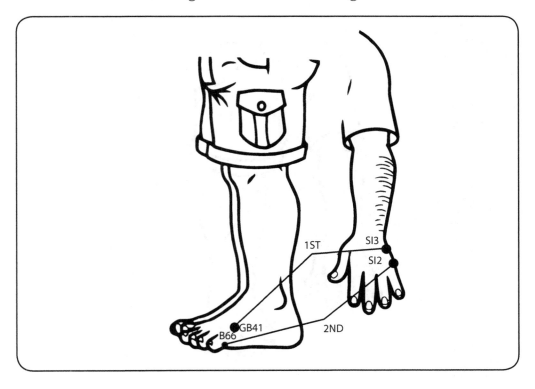

Fig,. 11.22 - Small Intestine Strengthening

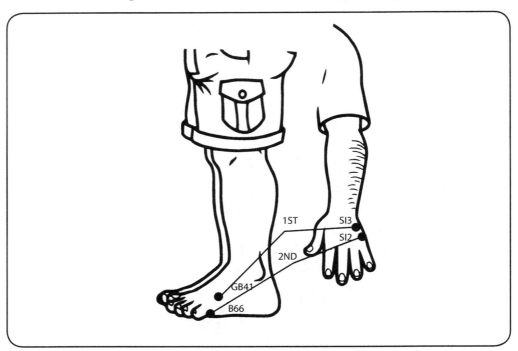

Fig. 11.23 - Small Intestine Sedating

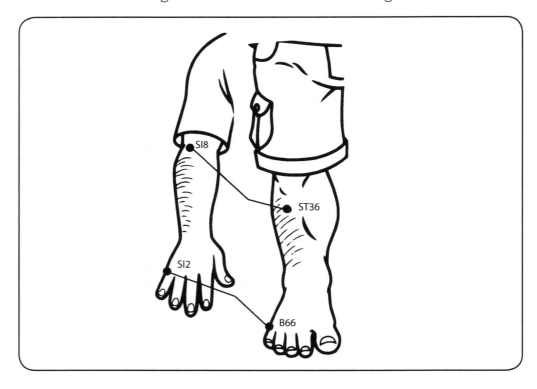

Fig. 11.24 - Bladder Strengthening

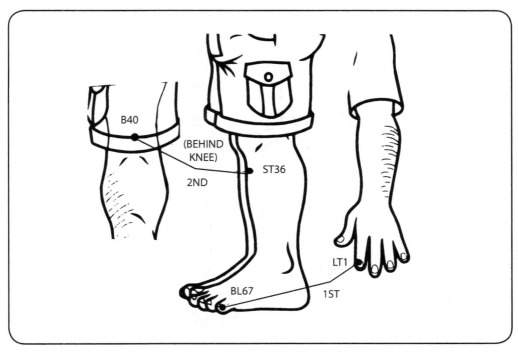

Fig. 11.25 - Bladder Sedating

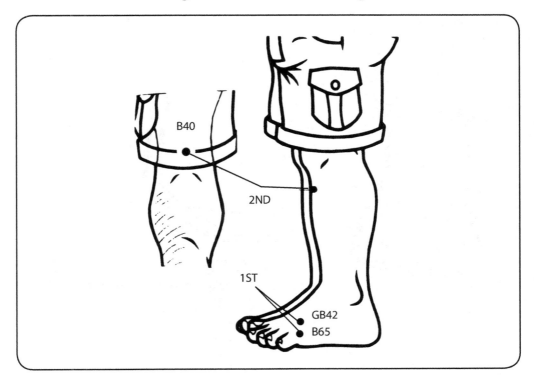

Fig. 11.26 - Kidney Strengthening

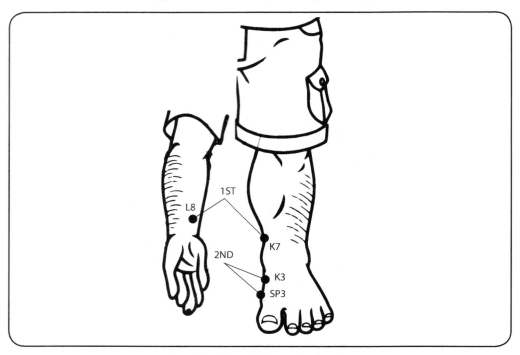

Fig. 11.27 - Kidney Sedating

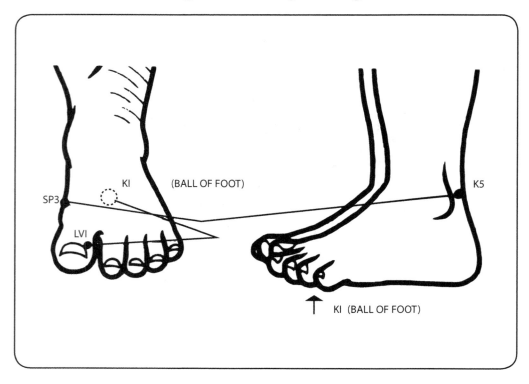

Fig. 11.28 - Circulation-Sex Strengthening

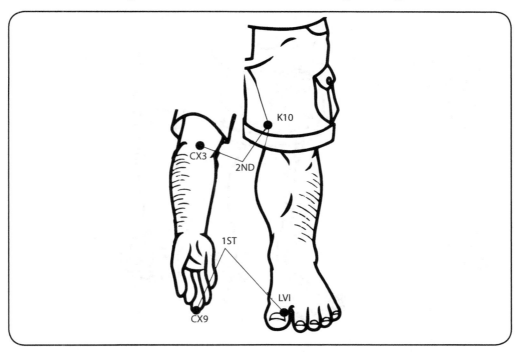

Fig. 11.29 - Circulation-Sex Sedating

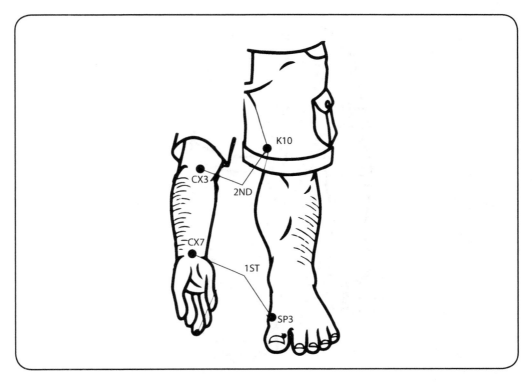

Fig. 11.30 - Triple Warmer Strengthening

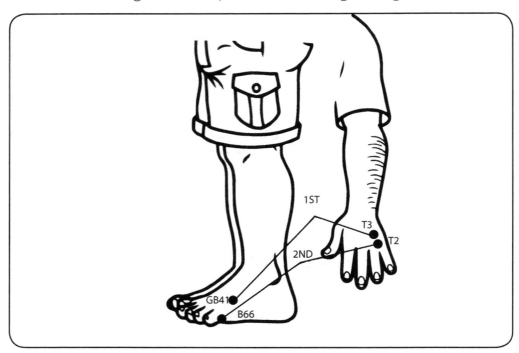

Fig. 11.31 - Triple Warmer Sedating

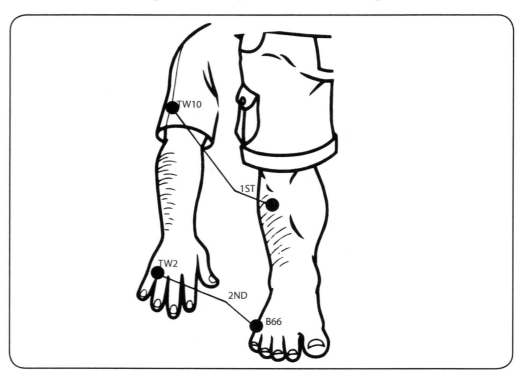

Fig. 11.32 - Gallbladder Strengthening

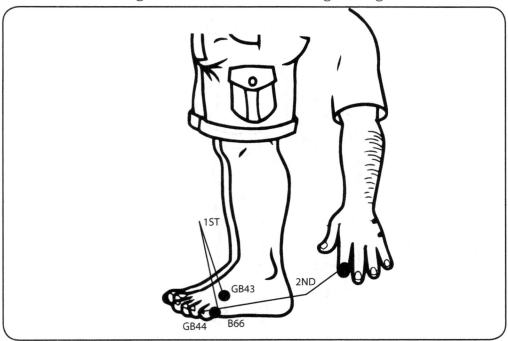

Fig. 11.33 - Gallbladder Sedating

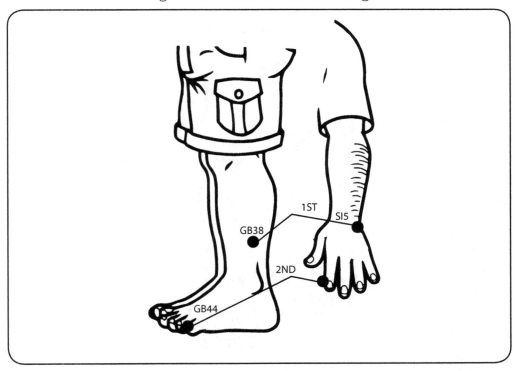

Fig. 11.34 - Liver Strengthening

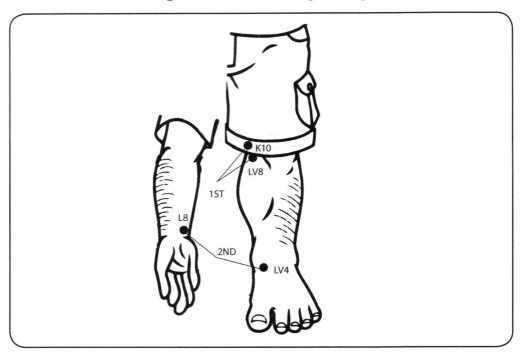

Fig. 11.35 - Liver Sedating

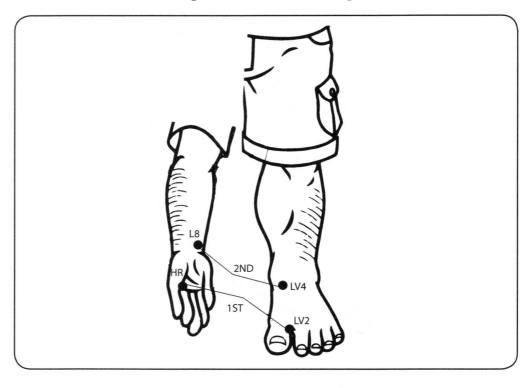

Fig. 11.36 - Lung Strengthening

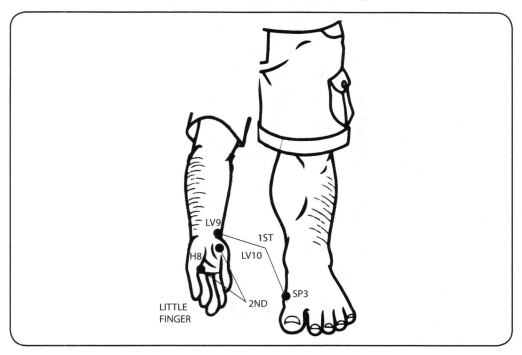

Fig. 11.37 - Lung Sedating

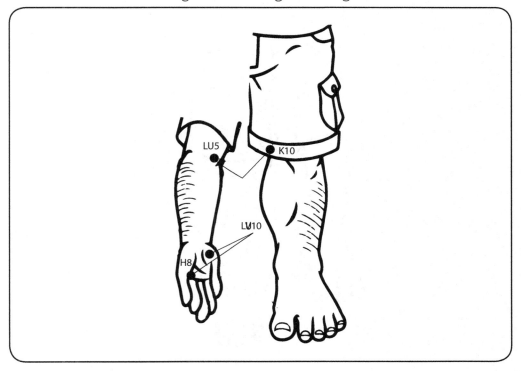

Fig. 11.38 - Large Intestine Strengthening

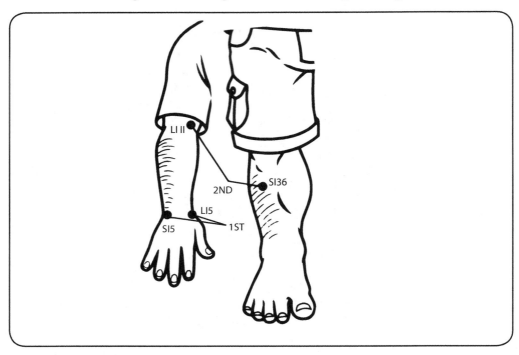

Fig. 11.39 - Large Intestine Sedating

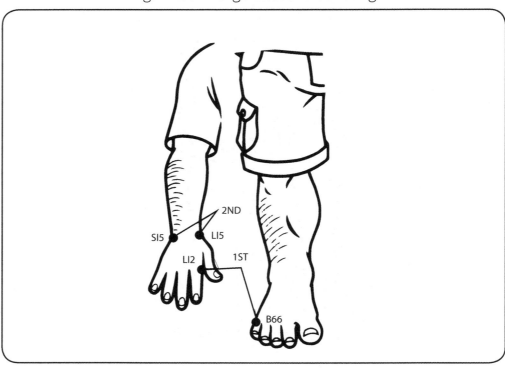

4. How to Hold Your Neurovascular Points

Neurovasculars govern what happens to blood and energy under stress. As well as being all over the head, they are also behind the knees, and in the center of the throat.

To hold the neurovasculars, you need to hold two sets of neurovascular points simultaneously: i) the main neurovasculars, which are located on the forehead, PLUS ii) the specific neurovascular point(s) that are associated with each particular meridian, and its related meridian.

Gently place your fingers on the relevant points, and then hold for up to five minutes, or until you feel a pulse, or some distinct 'lessening' or movement in your emotional intensity. *(See page 231 for more details about holding the neurovasculars).*

THE MAIN NEUROVASCULAR POINTS

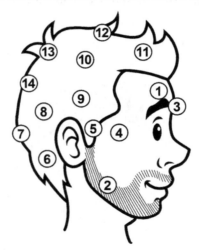

1. The main stress neurovascular points
2. Stomach
3. Bladder
4. Kidney
5. Triple Warmer
6. The main stress lymphatic points
7. Kidney
8. Circulation - X
9. Spleen
10. Large Intestine; Small Intestine; Kidney; Circulation - X
11. LIver
12. Lungs; Heart; Central; Liver; Gallbladder
13. Spleen
14. Triple Warmer

The Meridian Wheel

Each meridian usually has its own 'peak time,' a two-hour slot when its flow is particularly strong, or particularly weak. As Central Meridian is a 'global' meridian affecting the whole person, its peak time is generally at night, particularly around midnight. Governing Meridian, the other 'global' meridian, peaks in the day, around noon.

The energy in each meridian should be especially strong at its 'time of day.' If it's weak at that time, then it's clearly not getting the energetic juice it needs.

You can also diagnose what meridians may be blocked or unbalanced by seeing whether your symptoms show up at a particular time of day. For example, if the shooting pains in your legs tend to worsen between 3-5 pm, that could be a key indication that the Bladder Meridian is involved.

The Meridian Flow Wheel

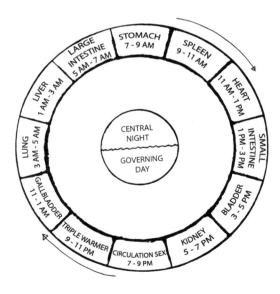

Working With the Triple Warmer Meridian

In all instances when working with weak or blocked meridians, the best place to start is by sedating Triple Warmer, as it will then shoot energy back to the areas and emotions that are weak or blocked.

Note: If you start working with the Triple Warmer Meridian on a regular basis, be sure to also strengthen your Spleen Meridian, to ensure that you still have enough pep and vitality. Frequently sedating Triple Warmer without also strengthening Spleen can sometimes weaken your energy system, leading to feelings of lethargy, sadness and depression.

Energy Testing Triple Warmer

You can do a very easy energy test to see if Triple Warmer is in 'overwhelm' mode. Simply cup your palm gently over the ear of the person being tested, and ask them to hold their hand out in front of them, palm open and palm down.

Tell them to 'resist' the pressure you're about to apply to their arm, then, using two fingers, gently press down on their wrist, as you cup their ear with your other hand. If Triple Warmer is freaking out, they won't be able to keep their arm up.

Retest after doing some of the exercises below, to see if you managed to get Triple Warmer to calm down.

What you can do to get Triple Warmer to calm down

As you learned in the chapter on meridians, understanding the mechanics of what's actually going on inside you energetically when you fly off the handle or start to feel very anxious and weak, is already a huge part of being able to resolve the emotional issue. So many people tell us that we just need to 'try' to stop getting angry, or to 'think positive,' and that will take care of the fear, (or whatever negative emotion you're having a problem with) but that's only half the solution.

Anger and fear are physiological reactions that God has programmed into our physical bodies via the subconscious reactions that occur in our so-called 'primitive' brain. When you are missing this part of the puzzle, you can work on your anger for years, and even pray about your anger for years, and still get taken by surprise when a situation or person presses your subconscious 'anger' button and you react like King Kong.

As previously mentioned, if you only try to use the Energy Medicine techniques described here to deal with your emotional and physical issues, without talking to God about them as well, either it won't work very well, or it won't carry on working, or the problem will just pop up in some other area of your life, because you didn't uproot it spiritually, and get God involved in the process.

For things to really move, you need to combine talking to God with energy-moving techniques to take Triple Warmer off alert, and to start balancing out the other meridians. The following techniques are commonly used in Energy Medicine (as taught by Donna Eden) and also Energy Psychology. The more you use these techniques, the calmer you'll start to feel, even in stressful situations that would usually get you instantly scared, angry or irritable.

A calm Triple Warmer plays a crucial function in maintaining good mental and physical health, so there's a lot of good reasons to give the following exercises a go.

TRIPLE WARMER TECHNIQUES

Technique One: Tap the 'fear' points on the hand

When you tap on the outside of the hand, between the joints of your ring and pinkie finger, you are sending an energy signal to your nervous system (i.e., Triple Warmer) that all is well, and that it doesn't have to be scared.

Start tapping when you are actively feeling the fear – i.e., the siren is going off, they are making cuts at work, your mother-in-law is coming for two months - and keep going until you feel the fear subside.

You can still think about the 'problem' or issue afterwards - it didn't zap it out of your memory banks - but you've disabled the stress response that makes you overreact or react unhelpfully.

Technique Two: The Triple Warmer 'smoothie'

This is working directly on the Triple Warmer Meridian, which goes from the temples, up behind the ears and down both arms to the ring finger (yes, THAT's why you get so many tension headaches...).

Put your fingers on your temples, and take a deep breath in. Exhale, and take your fingers up behind your ears, using some gentle pressure. Trace down behind your ears, down your neck, to your shoulders. Hang your hands on your neck for as long as it feels good, then drop your hands away.

Mentally, it helps to imagine yourself throwing all the worries away, when your hands drop.

The more you do the Smoothie, the more you'll calm down Triple Warmer, energetically.

Technique Three: Sedate Triple Warmer using acupressure points

This is the 'heavy artillery' of the Energy Medicine techniques to keep Triple Warmer calm. This works amazing with kids (or adults) who are too worried, anxious, angry or panicked to sleep. Simply hold the points (as described below) for five minutes, and the person should visibly relax, and feel much calmer, physically.

If you're going through a very taxing time, or you're feeling more angry, fearful or stressed than usual, you can hold these points three times a day (although you can hold them more without doing any damage to yourself, as one of the big benefits of acupressure is that it's completely non-invasive).

Otherwise, you should probably stick to holding them once a day, even when you're feeling calm and happy, to try and keep it that way. (Remember, the effects are cumulative. The more you do these procedures, the calmer you'll feel when the next big stress or problem hits.)

Technique Four: Hold the neurovasculars

Defusing Stress Emotions with the Neurovasculars

Few things feel worse than the feeling you get when you've just been hit by a massive dose of fear, shame, guilt or criticism. All the blood rushes away from your brain, and you can literally feel like the floor is falling away from you.

All of us respond to these extreme stress emotions of being 'assaulted' or 'attacked' in different ways: one person will freeze in place, another will react with rage, still another will literally run away or mentally switch off (which is essentially the same thing).

Again, these are knee-jerk reactions that are governed by our primitive brain, and they often tend to catch us by surprise. We start reacting emotionally before our conscious brain is even aware of what's going on.

So what can we do, to try to discharge our extreme negative reactions? Let me introduce you to a very simple Energy Medicine technique called **holding the neurovasculars.**

The main neurovascular points on your head are the bits of your forehead that jut out, a centimeter or two above both your eyebrows. To defuse any overwhelming feelings of stress, shame, guilt, anxiety or fear, simply gently hold these points for between 2 to 5 minutes, and continue to think about the 'stressful thought,' person, situation or experience.

Within five minutes, the negative emotional reaction to the stressful thought should either be completely neutralized, or so far reduced that you can function again.

How does this work?

Again, very simply, when you hold those points, you bring the blood back into your forehead, which is the place where a person can think rationally, using their higher mental and spiritual faculties. When we get stressed, up to 80% of the blood leaves this area, pulled away by the hypothalamus (and Triple Warmer) to fuel the 'fight or flight' response.

That energy is either going to your legs, so you can run away, or it's getting you ready to punch someone's face in. When you gently hold your neurovascular points, however, you encourage the blood to flow back into your thinking faculties, and away from your emotional knee-jerk reactions.

Technique Five: The karate chop instant calmer

This is a deceptively simple, but very effective Energy Psychology technique to stop a panic, rage or anxiety attack in its tracks. Simply repeatedly tap the side of the hand known as the 'karate chop,' until you start to feel like your feelings are 'depressurizing.'

In Energy Psychology, this is usually used as part of a tapping routine, and is usually paired with a phrase, or some wording. But it works well to directly 'depressurize' stress emotions even when it's done 'mindlessly' - and when someone is in the middle of being overwhelmed by their negative emotions, they usually can't think straight in any case.

Appendix 2

Guide to Dissolving Your Emotional Blocks

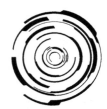

How to use this Guide:

The 'Talk to God' approach to dissolving emotional blocks and disconnecting your subconscious 'buttons' or triggers revolves around three things:

1. Get God involved in the process.

2. Identify what the negative emotion actually is, and what situations, circumstances, relationships or beliefs need to change, in order for the block to disappear.

3. Release the block energetically, by using specific Energy Medicine and Energy Psychology techniques.

Over the following pages, you'll learn how to apply these three steps to specific emotional blockages and issues.

Note: The online version of this Guide contains a number of embedded links for how to do the Tapas Acupressure Technique (TAT) pose, which is a very popular, effective and easy-to-use Energy Psychology technique. You can access the Guide at: www.jemi.website.

ANGER

1. Get God involved. Start a discussion based on the following ideas:

- Why am I angry?

- Who, or what, is making me angry?

- What good thing is hidden in my anger?

- What do You want me to change, fix or acknowledge, in order for the anger to disappear?

2. Identify what's triggering the anger.

Answering the following questions will help you to get more in touch with your actual feeling of anger.

- How would you describe your anger? (Volcanic, enraged, furious, murderous, etc.)

- How do you react to your anger? (Do you feel like you're going to explode? Lash out? Scream? Do you get sarcastic and insulting, or do you react with more passive aggression?)

- Where do you feel the anger in your body? (Clenched fists? Tight chest? Pounding in the temples?)

- When do you feel angry? (Who, or what, routinely triggers it?)

- What is it about the situations you find yourself in that makes you feel so angry?

- Why do you want to hold on to your anger?

- What good things will happen when you let go of your anger?

Whenever you feel you've hit an emotional 'charge,' or blockage, use the Tapas Acupressure Technique (TAT) to defuse it, as follows:

I.   State the problem:

■ 'I'm murderously angry.'

■ 'I can't express my anger in a healthy way.'

■ 'My chest gets really tight, whenever I'm angry.'

■ 'Being forced to attend family get-togethers makes me feel angry.'

■ 'I'm so angry that I feel powerless.'

■ 'I'm holding on to my anger, because it's protecting me.'

■ 'I don't want to let go of my anger...'

II. Go through the 7 Tapas Acupressure Technique (TAT) steps, focusing on one problem at a time.

III. Make a note of any insights you gained - but know that God is now healing the source of the problem, so relax and let Him do His thing.

3.   Dissolve the block at the energetic level.

The meridians to work with for anger:

Liver:	*Sedate to reduce beating yourself up, self-hatred or anger at the self*
Gallbladder:	*Sedate to reduce anger at others*
Spleen:	*Strengthen, to encourage feelings of compassion*
Triple Warmer:	*Sedate to lessen the 'fight' part of the fight-or-flight reaction*

ANXIETY

1.   Get God involved. Start a discussion based on the following ideas:

- Why am I anxious?

- Who, or what, is making me anxious?

- What good thing is hidden in my anxiety?

- What do You want me to change, fix or acknowledge, in order for the anxiety to disappear?

2.   Identify what's triggering the anxiety.

Answering the following questions will help you to get more in touch with your actual feeling of anxiety.

- How would you describe your anxiety? (Panic, paralysis, etc.)

- How do you react to your anxiety? (Freeze in place? Reach for the chocolate, Gameboy, or whiskey? Start thinking obsessively?)

- Where do you feel the anxiety in your body? (Heart racing? Tension headache? Butterflies in your stomach?)

- When do you feel anxious? (Who or what routinely triggers it?)

- What is it about the situations you find yourself in that makes you feel so anxious?

- Why do you want to hold on to your anxiety?

- What good things will happen when you let go of your anxiety?

Whenever you feel you've hit an emotional 'charge' or blockage, use the Tapas Acupressure Technique (TAT) to defuse it as follows:

I.   State the problem:

- "I'm paralyzed with anxiety."

- "My feelings of anxiety are leading to a lot of negative behaviors."

- "I feel really ill when I get anxious."

- "Being yelled at makes me feel really anxious."

- "I'm anxious that I'm doing something wrong, and I'm going to get punished for it."

- "I'm holding on to my anxiety, because it's keeping me in line."

■ "I don't want to let go of my anxiety, it's like an old friend."

II. Go through the 7 Tapas Acupressure Technique (TAT) steps, focusing on one problem at a time.

III. Make a note of any insights you gained - but know that God is now healing the source of the problem, so relax and let Him do His thing.

3.   Dissolve the block at the energetic level.

The meridians to work with for anxiety:

Kidney: *Sedate to dissipate deep-seated fear*

Bladder: *Sedate to disperse futility, despair or pessimism*

Spleen: *Strengthen to boost your joy*

Triple Warmer: *Sedate to lessen overwhelming fear that 'something bad is going to happen'*

BEATING YOURSELF UP

1.   Get God involved. Start a discussion based on the following ideas:

■ Why am I beating myself up?

■ What happened to trigger this 'beating myself up' fit?

■ Why am I finding it so hard to accept that You're running the world, God, not me?

■ What do You want me to change, fix or acknowledge, in order for the beating myself up stuff to disappear?

2.   Identify what's triggering the 'beating yourself up.'

■ How would you describe your 'beating yourself up'? (Guilty, obsessive, blaming, angry, worried, etc.)

■ How do you react to your 'beating yourself up'? (Do you start second-guessing yourself? Replaying conversations or situations obsessively in your head? Make excuses for yourself, or other people? Turn to others for reassurance that you're really 'OK', etc.?)

■ Where do you feel the 'beating yourself up' in your body? (Empty pit in the stomach? Feeling of being squeezed in the chest? Drooping shoulders and hunched back?)

■ When do you start to beat yourself up? (Who or what routinely triggers it?)

■ What is it about the situations you find yourself in that makes you start beating yourself up? (Do you feel blamed? Responsible? Bad, etc.?)

■ Why do you want to continue beating yourself up?

■ What good things will happen when you stop beating yourself up?

Whenever you feel you've hit an emotional 'charge' or blockage, use the Tapas Acupressure Technique (TAT) to defuse it as follows:

I. State the problem:

■ "I feel terrible that I did [fill in the blank]."

■ "I can't stop going over what happened in my head."

■ "I feel like I've just been punched in the stomach."

■ "Whenever I'm around [name], I start beating myself up."

■ "I start beating myself up because I feel I'm to blame for [fill in the blank]."

■ "If I don't keep beating myself up, I'm scared I'll just let myself off the hook."

■ "I don't want to stop beating myself up..."

II. Go through the 7 Tapas Acupressure Technique (TAT) steps, focusing on one problem at a time.

III. Make a note of any insights you gained - but know that God is now healing the source of the problem, so relax and let Him do His thing.

3.   Dissolve the block at the energetic level.

The meridians to work with for beating yourself up:

Liver: *Sedate to stop beating yourself up, self-hatred, anger at the self*

Gallbladder: *Sedate to reduce anger at others*

Triple Warmer: *Sedate to lessen overwhelming feelings of fear that you're bad, or that you've done something wrong*

DEPRESSION

Note: Depression is a huge subject, and requires the sort of discussion that is beyond the scope of this course. You can download a free eBook called 'The Causes and Cures of Depression' on the JEMI website that will give you a lot of detailed information and tools for what may be making you depressed, and how to pull out of it.

Read that book, then apply the following steps to the ideas you've just learned:

1.   Get God involved. Start a discussion based on the following ideas:

■ Why am I depressed?

■ Who, or what, is making me depressed?

■ What good thing is hidden in my depression?

■ What do You want me to change, fix or acknowledge, in order for the depression to disappear?

2.   Identify what's triggering the depression.

Note: Read 'The Causes and Cures of Depression' before answering the following questions!

- How would you describe your depression? (Feel dead inside, feel like you have no life, no energy, don't want to be alive anymore, etc.)

- How do you react to your depression? (Stay in bed all day? Cry? Avoid social interactions? Start beating yourself up?)

- Where do you feel the depression in your body? (Heaviness, pain, emptiness)

- When do you feel depressed? (Who or what routinely triggers it?)

- What is it about the situations you find yourself in that makes you feel so depressed?

- Why do you want to hold on to your depression?

- What good things will happen when you let go of your depression?

Whenever you feel you've hit an emotional 'charge' or blockage, use the Tapas Acupressure Technique (TAT) to defuse it as follows:

I. State the problem:

- "I don't want to be alive anymore."

- "I'm so depressed I can't even get out of bed."

- "My body feels so heavy, even standing up is an effort."

- "I don't care about anything, or anyone."

- "I'm holding on to my depression, because I'm scared to let go of it."

- "I don't want to stop feeling depressed..."

II. Go through the 7 Tapas Acupressure Technique (TAT) steps, focusing on one problem at a time.

III. Make a note of any insights you gained - but know that God is now healing the source of the problem, so relax and let Him do His thing.

3.   Dissolve the block at the energetic level.

The meridians to work with for depression (but only once you've made coming out of the homolateral energy state your priority):

Kidney:	*Strengthen to boost your innate life force*
Bladder:	*Sedate to dissipate futility, despair or pessimism*
Spleen:	*Strengthen to boost your joy*
Triple Warmer:	*Sedate to encourage your energy to 'unfreeze'*

What is the 'Homolateral Energy State'?

Normally, the energy in your body crosses over in many different ways and permutations. When your body's energy goes into the homolateral energy state, that means that instead of crossing over, your energy is now flowing up and down your body, in parallel lines.

When this happens, it reduces your energy by more than 50%, making it much harder for you to get or stay well, and contributes greatly to the listless, heavy, frozen feeling that often characterizes the state of clinical depression.

It's very easy to get the energy crossing over again (you'll find details of how to do this in "The Causes and Cures of Depression Pocket Guide," published by The Matronita Press, but it often takes a bit of perseverance to maintain the energy crossover, long-term.

DESPAIR

1. Get God involved. Start a discussion based on the following ideas:

■ Why do I feel so despairing?

■ Who, or what, is making me despair that things can never change or improve?

■ What good thing is hidden in my despair?

■ What do You want me to change, fix or acknowledge, in order for the despair to disappear?

2.   Identify what's triggering the despair.

■ How would you describe your despair? (Emptiness, grief, past caring, etc.)

■ How do you react to your despair? (Won't try new things, cynicism, try to spoil things for others)

■ Where do you feel the despair in your body? (Heavy head? Heavy heart? Backaches? Slumped posture?)

■ When do you feel despairing? (Who or what routinely triggers it?)

■ What is it about the situations you find yourself in that makes you feel so despairing?

■ Why do you want to hold on to your despair?

■ What good things will happen when you let go of your despair?

Whenever you feel you've hit an emotional 'charge' or blockage, use the Tapas Acupressure Technique (TAT) to defuse it as follows:

I.   State the problem:

■ "I've given up."

■ "I don't believe things can ever change or improve."

■ "I feel so cynical and bitter."

■ "Things never work out for me'."

■ "I feel that God hates me."

■ "I don't want to try anymore, because I can't stand the disappointment when it doesn't work out."

■ "I don't want to let go of my despair, because then I'll have to start trying things again, and they're only going to end in failure."

■ "I don't want to stop feeling despairing..."

II. Go through the 7 Tapas Acupressure Technique (TAT) steps, focusing on one problem at a time.

III. Make a note of any insights you gained - but know that God is now healing the source of the problem, so relax and let Him do His thing.

3. Dissolve the block at the energetic level.

The meridians to work with for despair:

Kidney:	*Sedate to disperse feelings of isolation*
Bladder:	*Sedate to dissolve futility, despair or pessimism*
Stomach:	*Sedate to reduce everyday worry and stress*
Spleen:	*Strengthen to boost your joy*
Heart:	*Strengthen to help you love yourself again*

EMPTINESS

1. Get God involved. Start a discussion based on the following ideas:

- Why do I feel so empty?

- What would really make me feel 'filled up'?

- What good thing is hidden in this emptiness?

- What do You want me to change, fix or acknowledge, in order for the emptiness to disappear?

2. Identify what's triggering the 'emptiness.'

- How would you describe your emptiness?

- How do you react to your emptiness? (Go into hiding? Fill it with food? Drown it with work deadlines? Spend hours on Facebook?)

- Where do you feel the emptiness in your body?

- When do you feel empty? (Who or what routinely triggers it?)

- What is it about the situations you find yourself in that makes you feel so empty?

- Why do you want to hold on to your emptiness?

- What good things will happen when you let go of your emptiness?

Whenever you feel you've hit an emotional 'charge' or blockage, use the Tapas Acupressure Technique (TAT) to defuse it as follows:

I.   State the problem:

- "I feel I don't exist."

- "I feel disconnected from everything, and everyone."

- "Nothing ever really fills me up."

- "I eat obsessively to try to fill the emptiness I feel."

- "I don't believe anyone really cares about me."

- "My ideas / thoughts / opinions don't matter."

- "I don't want to let go of my emptiness..."

II. Go through the 7 Tapas Acupressure Technique (TAT) steps, focusing on one problem at a time.

III. Make a note of any insights you gained - but know that God is now healing the source of the problem, so relax and let Him do His thing.

3.   Dissolve the block at the energetic level.

The meridians to work with for emptiness:

Kidney: *Sedate to reduce toxic shame, strengthen to boost your will to live*

Bladder: *Sedate to disperse futility, despair or pessimism*

Lungs: *Sedate to clear grief, disappointment and aloofness*

Large Intestine: *Sedate to let other people into your life*

Spleen: *Strengthen to boost your joy and self-compassion*

Heart: *Strengthen to help you love yourself more*

FEAR - SEE ANXIETY

GUILT

1. Get God involved. Start a discussion based on the following ideas:

- Why do I feel guilty?

- Who, or what, is making me feel guilty?

- What good thing is hidden in my guilt feelings?

- What do You want me to change, fix or acknowledge, in order for the guilt to disappear?

2. Identify what's triggering the guilty feeling.

Answering the following questions will help you to get more in touch with your actual feeling of guilt.

- How would you describe your guilt? (Brain-freeze, panic, anxiety)

- How do you react to your guilt? (Go overboard trying to apologize? Try to buy people off? Beat yourself up? Blame others? Try to ignore it? Get angry?)

- Where do you feel the guilt in your body? (Nausea? Headache? Pain?)

- When do you feel guilty? (Who, or what, routinely triggers it?)

- What is it about the situations you find yourself in that makes you feel so guilty?

- Why do you want to hold on to your guilt?

- What good things will happen when you let go of your guilt?

Whenever you feel you've hit an emotional 'charge' or blockage, use the Tapas Acupressure Technique (TAT) to defuse it as follows:

I. State the problem:

- "I feel guilty all the time."

- "I feel guilty every time I have to say 'no.'"

- "I feel like a bad person."

- "I feel like I always have to fix other people's problems."

- "I people-please all the time, so I won't feel bad about myself."

- "I feel so bad when I make a mistake, I can't deal with it."

- "I'm holding on to my guilt, because God wants me to feel bad about what I did (or didn't do)."

- "I don't want to let go of my guilt..."

II. Go through the 7 Tapas Acupressure Technique (TAT) steps, focusing on one problem at a time.

III. Make a note of any insights you gained - but know that God is now healing the source of the problem, so relax and let Him do His thing.

3. Dissolve the block at the energetic level.

The meridians to work with for anxiety:

Kidney: *Sedate to dispel toxic shame*

Liver: *Sedate to dispel guilt and self-hatred*

Spleen: *Strengthen to boost your joy and self-compassion*

Triple Warmer: *Sedate to reduce overwhelming fear that 'something bad is going to happen'*

HATRED - SEE ANGER

INDECISION

1. Get God involved. Start a discussion based on the following ideas:

- Why am I so indecisive?

- Who, or what, is making me indecisive?

- What good thing is hidden in my indecision?

- What do You want me to change, fix or acknowledge, in order for me to become more decisive?

2.   Identify what's triggering the indecision.

- How would you describe your indecision? (Panic, paralysis, obsessive thinking, etc.)

- How do you react to your indecision? (Avoid decisions, make them impulsively, get others to decide for you)

- Where do you feel the indecision in your body? (Brain fuzz? Churning stomach?)

- When do you feel indecisive? (Who, or what, routinely triggers it?)

- What is it about the situations you find yourself in that makes you feel so indecisive? (Who are you worried about pleasing? What will happen if you don't make the right choice?)

- Why do you want to hold on to your indecision?

- What good things will happen when you let go of your indecision?

Whenever you feel you've hit an emotional 'charge' or blockage, use the Tapas Acupressure Technique (TAT) to defuse it as follows:

I.   State the problem:

- "I can't make any decisions."

- "I feel very anxious when I have to make a decision."

- "I feel really ill when I have to make a choice."

- "I'm worried I'm going to do something wrong."

- "I don't want to be blamed for making the wrong decision."

- "I'm holding on to my indecision, as then I don't have to take any responsibility for what happens."

- "I like being indecisive..."

II. Go through the 7 Tapas Acupressure Technique (TAT) steps, focusing on one problem at a time.

III. Make a note of any insights you gained - but know that God is now healing the source of the problem, so relax and let Him do His thing.

3.   Dissolve the block at the energetic level.

The meridians to work with for indecision:

Stomach:	*Sedate to dispel anxiety, worry and pessimism*
Small Intestine:	*Sedate to dissolve confusion and doubt, strengthen to promote decisiveness*
Spleen:	*Strengthen to boost your self-compassion*
Triple Warmer:	*Sedate to reduce overwhelming fear that 'something bad is going to happen'*

LONELINESS - SEE EMPTINESS

NERVOUSNESS - SEE ANXIETY

PANIC

1.   Get God involved. Start a discussion based on the following ideas:

- Why am I panicking?

- Who, or what, is making me panic?

- What good thing is hidden in my feelings of panic?

- What do You want me to change, fix or acknowledge, in order for the panic to disappear?

2. Identify what's triggering the panic

Answering the following questions will help you to get more in touch with your actual feeling of panic.

- How would you describe your panic? (Can't think, start yelling, can't breathe, etc.)

- How do you react to your anxiety? (Feel like you're going to throw up, start snapping at others, make irrational decisions)

- Where do you feel the panic in your body? (Heart racing? Blurry vision? Butterflies in your stomach?)

- When do you feel panicked? (Who, or what, routinely triggers it?)

- What is it about the situations you find yourself in that makes you feel so panicky?

- Why do you want to hold on to your panic?

- What good things will happen when you let go of your panic?

Whenever you feel you've hit an emotional 'charge' or blockage, use the Tapas Acupressure Technique (TAT) to defuse it as follows:

I. State the problem:

- "The thought of starting something new makes me panic."

- "I panic whenever I feel I've done something wrong."

- "I feel like I'm going to throw up."

- "I start panicking whenever I think about what could go wrong."

- "I hate the feeling that I'm not in control."

- "I don't want to stop panicking..."

II. Go through the 7 Tapas Acupressure Technique (TAT) steps, focusing on one problem at a time.

III. Make a note of any insights you gained - but know that God is now healing the source of the problem, so relax and let Him do His thing.

3.   Dissolve the block at the energetic level.

The meridians to work with for panic:

Circulation-Sex: *Sedate to dissipate over-commitment and frustration*

Small Intestine: *Strengthen to increase ability to make a decision calmly*

Stomach: *Sedate to dissolve worry, stress and pessimism*

Spleen: *Strengthen to boost your joy*

Large Intestine: *Sedate to reduce control-freak tendencies, inability to 'let go' of outcomes*

Triple Warmer: *Sedate to reduce overwhelming fear that 'something bad is going to happen'*

RAGE - SEE ANGER

RESENTMENT - SEE ANGER

SELF-HATRED - SEE BEATING YOURSELF UP

SHAME (TOXIC SHAME)

1.   Get God involved. Start a discussion based on the following ideas:

■ Why do I feel so ashamed?

■ Who, or what, is making me feel ashamed and worthless?

■ What good thing is hidden in my feelings of shame?

■ What do You want me to change, fix or acknowledge, in order for the shame to disappear?

2. Identify what's triggering the toxic shame.

■ How would you describe your toxic shame? (Feel like you want the floor to open up and swallow you, feel like you're 'bad,' feel like you're a disgusting human being, etc.)

■ How do you react to your toxic shame? (Try to numb the pain somehow? Throw your self into work or socializing? Sink into depression?)

■ Where do you feel the shame in your body? (Burning cheeks? Tightness in your chest? Feel like your head is going to explode?)

■ When do you feel ashamed or worthless? (Who, or what, routinely triggers it?)

■ What is it about the situations you find yourself in that makes you feel so ashamed and worthless?

■ Why do you want to hold on to your shame?

■ What good things will happen when you let go of your toxic shame?

Whenever you feel you've hit an emotional 'charge' or blockage, use the Tapas Acupressure Technique (TAT) to defuse it as follows:

I. State the problem:

■ "I feel like I'm scum."

■ "I feel like the world would be better off without me."

■ "I just make trouble, wherever I go."

■ "I'm broken, and I can't be fixed."

■ "Every time I do [fill in the blank], I feel terrible afterwards."

■ "After I speak to [fill in blank], I come away feeling so worthless."

■ "All the horrible things [fill in the blank] said about me are true'"

■ "Some of the people I love the most make me feel awful about myself."

■ "I can't stop feeling so worthless and bad."

II. Go through the 7 Tapas Acupressure Technique (TAT) steps, focusing on one problem at a time.

III. Make a note of any insights you gained - but know that God is now healing the source of the problem, so relax and let Him do His thing.

3. Dissolve the block at the energetic level.

The meridians to work with for toxic shame:

Kidney:	*Sedate to dissolve deep-seated fear, trauma and shame, strengthen to boost your will to live*
Bladder:	*Sedate to decrease futility, despair or pessimism*
Liver:	*Sedate to stop self-hatred and beating yourself up*
Spleen:	*Strengthen to boost your joy and self-compassion*
Heart:	*Strengthen to start liking yourself and overcome heartache*
Triple Warmer:	*Sedate to reduce overwhelming fear of being punished for doing (or being…) something 'wrong'*

WORRY

1. Get God involved. Start a discussion based on the following ideas:

- Why am I so worried?

- Who, or what, is making me worried?

- What good thing is hidden in my worry?

- What do You want me to change, fix or acknowledge, in order for the worry to disappear?

2. Identify what's triggering the worry.

- How would you describe your worry? (Feelings of stress, can't think, can't sleep, can't concentrate, over-analyzing everything)

- How do you react to your worry? (Start trying to control? Get angry and fragile? Disconnect from reality and space out?)

- Where do you feel the worry in your body? (Heart racing? Tension headache? Butterflies in your stomach?)

- When do you feel worry? (Who, or what, routinely triggers it?)

- What is it about the situations you find yourself in that makes you feel so worried?

- Why do you want to hold on to your worry?

- What good things will happen when you let go of your worry?

Whenever you feel you've hit an emotional 'charge' or blockage, use the Tapas Acupressure Technique (TAT) to defuse it as follows:

I.   State the problem:

- "I keep worrying about my finances."

- "Worrying about my finances is keeping me awake at night."

- "I'm so worried about how I'm going to pay off the credit card, it's starting to affect my appetite."

- "I'm worried I'm going to be blamed for things going wrong."

- "I'm worried that I'm going to feel terrible, if it doesn't turn out OK."

- "I feel if I worry about something, it won't happen."

- "I can't be happy, unless X happens (or doesn't happen)."

- "I don't want to stop worrying - it's the responsible thing to do."

II. Go through the 7 Tapas Acupressure Technique (TAT) steps, focusing on one problem at a time.

III. Make a note of any insights you gained - but know that God is now healing the source of the problem, so relax and let Him do His thing.

3.   Dissolve the block at the energetic level.

The meridians to work with for worry:

Kidney: *Sedate to dissolve deep-seated fear and trauma*

Bladder: *Sedate to dissipate futility, despair or pessimism*

Stomach:	*Sedate to reduce anxiety, worry and general stress*
Large Intestine:	*Sedate to dissolve inability to let go and stop controlling*
Spleen:	*Strengthen to boost your joy*
Triple Warmer:	*Sedate to reduce overwhelming fear that 'something bad is going to happen'*

Appendix 3

The 'Talk to God' Approach In Action - The Client Case Files

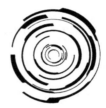

Esther's Broken Toe

Esther came in with a broken toe - her second within a year - and wanted to try to get a deeper understanding of why she seemed to keep breaking her toes, apparently for no reason.

In Chinese medicine, Kidney Meridian is associated with a bunch of various things in the body, but one of the main things it governs is bones. Kidney Meridian is considered to be the deepest energy meridian of the body, and it's also the repository of a person's will to live, or inner vitality.

What all this means, practically, is that when the energy in the Kidney Meridian is weak, a person is then much more susceptible to broken bones.

Knocks and scrapes that you'd ordinarily shrug off start to break you, literally, when the energy in Kidney Meridian is impaired, because your vital life force is very low, and you're physically and spiritually very weak.

One of the things I love the most about the Energy Medicine stuff is that it's really like a detective story, where you're trying to help each person to piece together all the different bits of their personal health puzzle.

The next thing Esther learned is that the main negative emotion that governs the Kidney Meridian is fear. Chronic or constant fear and anxiety is probably the single most damaging emotion a person can have.

Last year, Esther had been going through a really tough year. At the time she broke her toe for the second time, she'd just been through an extremely difficult period where her husband had been made redundant and money had gotten extremely tight.

Esther was feeling very scared about the future - about her family's finances and about her husband's plans to start up a new business - and most days, she was functioning on zero energy.

She literally felt emptied out at the soul level, like she had no more strength. Physically, she could still get up and do things and cook and walk, but mentally and emotionally, she'd passed 'exhausted' a long time ago. All the fear about 'what will be,' and about what had just happened, were draining away all her life force, leaving her Kidney Meridian really depleted.

Small wonder that Esther kept on breaking her toes!

Together, we worked out a plan of how to get Esther's energy and *joie de vivre* back up. Physically, I suggested that Esther should hold the acupressure strengthening and sedating points for Kidney Meridian, and that she should also sedate Triple Warmer (which was pressing the internal 'panic' button a bit too much) along with strengthening Spleen Meridian (which produces the 'happy juice' for us). I recommended doing this at least twice a day, until she started to feel her energy and mood improve.

Next, I suggested Esther should start talking to God for at least 5 minutes a day, so she wouldn't feel so alone in her struggles and afraid of the unknown. Remember, Kidney is weakened by fear and shame, and these are very hard emotions to shift if we haven't got God involved in the process.

The last thing was to encourage Esther to try to have more compassion for herself and the difficult situation she and her husband had just been through. (Remember, we need strong Spleen energy to have compassion for ourselves and others.) She was going to be strengthening her Spleen energetically by holding the acupressure points, but another way to strengthen Spleen is to slow down a bit, put some of the less urgent chores and demands on the back burner, and start to care for herself a little more.

Even though money was still very tight, I encouraged Esther to schedule a regular bubble bath, a coffee at a friend's, or even just a regular slot where she'd sit down every week, and do her nails, or paint a picture, do some gardening, or knit a scarf - whatever would feel like a nurturing, fulfilling experience for her.

To date, Esther hasn't had any more broken bones, she's starting to feel more physically replenished and stronger, which is also helping her to feel generally more confident and optimistic about life.

Adam's Bad Back

Adam is a fit man in his early forties who eats well, exercises, and hasn't been anywhere near a doctor for the last 20 years. Recently, he started to experience excruciating pains in his lower back, which were completely immobilizing him. He was having trouble sleeping, and could barely stand up, which meant he couldn't really work or pray.

The initial energy evaluation showed that Adam's Large Intestine and Kidney Meridians were out of balance. Like many men, Adam finds it difficult to talk about his emotions, or even to know what he's truly feeling. So God decided to help him out, by sending him a message he couldn't ignore or play down.

The Kidney Meridian is usually associated with fear; after some probing questions, it turned out Adam had recently gone through a tough patch in his life, and his belief that God was good, and that God was going to look after him, had been severely compromised. The rest of the session was spent using tapping (Energy Psychology) to remove Adam's negative beliefs about God, and then to build up Adam's belief that God really loved him. At the end of the two hour session, Adam started laughing deeply, and then burst into tears and said: "I really got it! God loves me!"

With that massive surprise revelation surfacing, he expected that his back would get much better, and for one day it did. But then, the pains started up again. This time, Adam went for a more 'practical' solution, and bought a new mattress. He slept on the new mattress for two days, but didn't see any improvement, so he came back for another session.

The pain had moved down from the original location in his back and now his legs were feeling very weak and shaky.

The Large Intestine Meridian, again, showed up as a problem area, so we focused on that. Large Intestine is connected to letting go of things, particularly toxic emotions.

After a brief discussion, it turned out that Adam had just had a couple of very close relationships turn sour, and as was his usual way, he hadn't dealt with the grief and emotional fallout; he'd just brushed it under his mental carpet and continued with his life.

Adam was shown the neurolymphatic points for the Large Intestine Meridian, and was told to massage them as firmly as he could stand, twice a day, to get all the waste material moving out, spiritually and physically.

He also had a treatment with a magnet to 'de-freeze' the Large Intestine Meridian that had 'frozen solid,' which means that the energy simply wasn't moving anywhere. The session ended with holding the acupressure points to sedate and then strengthen Adam's Large Intestine Meridian. His legs immediately felt better and less heavy.

In the three days following, Adam had a lot of 'stuff' move. Firstly, he had a day of feeling completely depressed and crushed, which wasn't fun, but was actually a necessary part of the process of owning and feeling his real emotions.

After he was reassured that it was all a normal, healthy part of the healing process, he stopped worrying that he was going to feel like this 'forever,' and just went with the flow. The next day, he felt much lighter and he regained more movement and flexibility in his back and legs.

That day, Adam went for a long walk, to talk to God about a number of things, and he came back having made some big decisions about how he wanted his life to change.

He wanted to go back to school to retrain as an architect, which had always been his life's dream. After discussing it with his wife, and getting her agreement, he took the drastic decision to cut down his work, so he could enroll for an architecture degree in his local college.

Adam was visibly happier, and lighter on his feet. But his back was still hurting.

Clearly, despite all the massive movement, something was still blocking his healing process. He came back for another session, and he was given treatment to promote deep relaxation and pain relief, and he was then told to wear a strip of lentils on two fingers overnight, where his spine was located in the Su Jok system [see the box]. As well as strengthening and healing the body, Seed Therapy is also an excellent diagnostic tool.

What is Su Jok?

Su Jok literally means 'hand and foot' in Korean, and it's a form of acupressure that was invented by Professor Jae Woo Park, back in the seventies.

Su Jok is based on the idea that the whole body is delineated on, and connected to, different parts of the human anatomy. This is a standard idea in many holistic therapies, including the diagnostic use of the tongue in traditional Chinese medicine, and Iridology, where the state of the eye reflects the health of the body.

Seed Therapy is an integral part of the Su Jok approach, where the healing power of seeds is applied to specific points of the patient's hand or foot, in the belief that the seed's innate energy will spark off a healing reaction in the part of the body that requires it.

The following morning, most of the lentils were cracked, showing that Adam's back was much weaker than he'd been letting on. (The lentils crack when the body has absorbed all of the energy they contain.)

Adam's voice was also sounding kind of swallowed and 'muffled,' which is a key sign that emotions are being blocked or repressed, often subconsciously. Adam was asked to rate the pain in his back, 10 being perfectly good health, and 0 being awful. He ranked the pain at a 3 or 4. Next, he was asked to look for and identify any negative emotion that he might be feeling. After a few seconds, he came back with 'worry.'

After a bit of probing, it turned out Adam was worrying that he wouldn't be able to keep up with the learning, that the whole 'architecture' thing would go sour, and that his decision to cut down work to switch careers would end in disaster.

Adam was coached through another 20 minute tapping session, this time focusing on replacing these negative worries with gratitude that he had the opportunity to follow his life's dream, and to trust God more that it was going to be exactly how it needed to be. At the end of his session, he ranked his back at a much healthier 7. The pain in his back continued to abate throughout the rest of the day.

Adam's back pain contained a profound lesson that the negative thoughts and emotions he was repressing were literally paralyzing him and sapping all of his strength and vitality. It took a couple of weeks to peel the onion, and get to the core of the problem, but now Adam knows that when his back twinges, or when he starts to feel himself stiffening and losing strength and flexibility, it's just a signal to go and track down the negative thought, worry or fear that was playing in his head. He can then uproot it and replace it with thoughts of trusting God and gratitude.

Matthew's Stomachache

Matthew had been experiencing pain in his lower abdomen for a couple of months. He'd been to the doctors and done all the tests, but nothing was showing up to explain it, so he decided to try something alternative. In this client case history, it quickly came up that Matthew had recently been through a very stressful time in his private life: the business that he'd been successfully running for more than two decades had hit a very rough patch and he'd been forced into bankruptcy.

Bankruptcy proceedings were still going on, and there was a strong possibility that Matthew would be forced to sell his family home to cover his debts, stressful circumstances by any means. Could it be connected to his abdominal pain? Matthew was a long distance client, so the usual hands-on Energy Medicine techniques couldn't be used, so I decided to work with Energy Psychology techniques.

Energy Psychology taps various points on the body, corresponding to the ends of the 14 energy meridians, to help release trapped energy, emotions, and pain. It can be a very effective technique, and can blast through some very deep-seated issues in just a session or two.

There are various ways of tapping, but Matthew was familiar with one of the most popular, called Emotional Freedom Technique (EFT). (You can learn the EFT routine for yourself at: www.emofree.com.)

I instructed Matthew to start tapping on the abdominal discomfort, which Matthew initially rated at a 6 or 7. EFT usually moves pretty fast, but after a few rounds of tapping, the stomachache was still at a 5 and didn't want to budge. This usually means one of two things: either, that there is a psychological reversal involved, i.e., there's a subconscious reason why the client wants to hang on to the problem, OR that there are other, deeper, aspects of the problem that haven't yet surfaced.

I asked Matthew if he'd ever had this sort of stomachache before. He thought for a moment, then in amazement, he told me that he'd had a very similar stomachache some 30-something years earlier, when he was 10. I asked him what had been going on in his life at that point and, still amazed, Matthew told me that his father's business had gone bust around that time, and the family had been forced to sell their home, as a result.

"How did you feel about that, as a 10-year-old?" I asked him.

"Terrible. My mother was depressed about it for years and my father just sort of collapsed in on himself after that. You couldn't talk to him. I felt like I lost everything I had in one shot: home, money, parents - everything."

I asked Matthew to rate his stomachache: it had shot up to a 9. We started tapping on the stomachache again, and again it came down a little, but then got stuck again. Something else was blocking our progress. Tapping is half mechanical, and half complete Heavenly help. So many times, it's happened to me that I've got stuck up a dead end with a client, and then God sends me a crucial piece of the puzzle as a gift. That's what happened now.

I asked Matthew how he felt, now that he was in a very similar situation to his father. After a few seconds' silence, he started crying.

To cut a very long story short, Matthew had never forgiven his father for his failures, and had sworn to himself, as a 10-year-old boy, that he was NEVER going to make the same mistakes with his life, and with his family. That harsh 10-year-old view of things had been governing Matthew, subconsciously, ever since. It had pushed him to be an overachiever, it had made him a workaholic and it had made him hate his father.

Now, God had put the adult Matthew in almost exactly the same situation, through no fault of his own, and his 10-year-old self was furious at Matthew for 'turning into his father.' One of the main things I asked Matthew to tap on a lot was the phrase:

"Even though I'm a failure, just like my father, I still love, accept and forgive myself unconditionally."

Matthew next realized that he also had to forgive his father, and let go of his 30-year-old resentment and hurt. If he didn't, he could see he was going to continue secretly hating *himself*, with big repercussions for his health and his state of mind.

By the end of that very intense session, the stomachache had gone and Matthew was feeling calmer inside than he had for years. But he also knew he had a lot of homework to do. First, he knew he had to make peace with his father, and to truly accept that his father had done the best he could, when his business failed.

Every time the thought that he, Matthew, was a failure 'just like his dad' popped into his head, he was to use EFT to forgive and accept himself, and his father. The other thing Matthew had to work on was his belief that God was running the world, and that everything that happened, both with his father's failed business and with his own, was truly for the best.

This can only really be done via regularly talking to God, so Matthew made a commitment to start talking to God for 10 minutes every day, and to take it up from there.

The stomachache, painful and uncomfortable as it was, really was a present from God, to help Matthew to finally forgive his father, and to help him go easier on himself and let God into his life more.

Matthew's Stomachache, Part II

You'll recall that Matthew had a stomachache as a result of some complicated emotions resulting from his imminent bankruptcy, and the bad memories it brought up from when his father lost his business when Matthew was a child.

Emotional Freedom Technique (EFT), or tapping, gave Matthew some big insights into his physical illness, and the spiritual and emotional actions he had to take to resolve it. The stomachache went away, but a couple of months later, it resurfaced.

This is not an unusual phenomenon. It doesn't necessarily mean that the original problem is back, because once the 'issue,' whatever it is, is resolved at its root in the soul, it's gone for good.

But what can often happen is that some previous symptoms can resurface, as God gets us ready to tackle the next layer down of the problem or issue. And that's exactly what happened with Matthew. I had a suspicion that the stomach was hiding something big, emotionally.

I had Matthew draw a mind-map, with the word 'stomach' in a box in the center. Then, I asked him to write anything and everything that came to mind, without censoring it, connected to the word 'stomach.' A couple of minutes later, he'd come up with the following list:

- Dark

- Bloated

- Black Hole

- Gas

- Icky

- Air

- Juices

- Fat

- Food

These are nearly all negative words. I asked Matthew to close his eyes and put his hands on his stomach, to get in touch with it for a few seconds. Next, I asked him to talk to his stomach, and ask it what it was trying to communicate to him. (This is a common psychotherapy technique called a Gestalt dialogue - but anyone can do this themselves, without any special training.)

The stomach told Matthew that he didn't have to hate himself. Matthew was surprised, first of all that his stomach was really telling him things, and also that it appeared to be pretty intelligent and clued-in. We continued.

After a few more minutes of Gestalt dialogue, Matthew's stomach had told him that he was eating junk food to try and make himself feel better, instead of just liking himself more. It also told him that he was nervous about making mistakes and doing things wrong (connected to what had surfaced earlier, about 'being a failure, just like his dad') and that's what was making him feel ill.

I instructed Matthew to ask his stomach what, in particular, he was nervous about right now. The answer came back very quickly: Things had been left up in the air with Matthew's former business partner. The business partner hadn't acted in a 100% correct way, and Matthew hadn't paid him money that otherwise was clearly owed to him, when the business dissolved. Matthew was in a quandary, and didn't know what to do about it all.

Whenever people are living a lie, or telling lies, even subconsciously, the stomach (and everything associated with it) is usually the place that's going to be directly affected. The good news is that telling the truth usually solves the spiritual problems affecting the stomach at their root, with immediate effect.

After some discussion, Matthew acknowledged that he knew that the truth was that he should pay his former business partner what he owed him, but he hadn't wanted to from fear of 'making a mistake' or being taken for a ride (again, connected to his fear of failure).

The stomach / solar plexus area is also the physical home of the ego. What we want, or what we feel is in our best interests, can sometimes clash with 'truth,' as it did here. Once the penny dropped that Matthew had to pay his business partner, he felt immediately better.

The stomachache reduced 90%. We ended the session with a visualization, where I asked Matthew to picture his stomach being filled up with the light of truth - God's truth - a kind, loving, warm, healing light, as opposed to a harsh Alcatraz-type spotlight.

The session ended with Matthew feeling much happier and more energetic, if still a little nervous about making the call to his former partner.

Sarah's ADHD

Sarah's mother brought her to me after Sarah's school forced her to undergo an evaluation for ADHD. The school psychologist was 'encouraging' Sarah's mother to put her daughter on Ritalin, but Sarah's mother was completely opposed to the use of drugs for children, and she also didn't believe that the ADHD diagnosis was accurate. After all, even though Sarah was 6 and still couldn't read, she could sit for hours being read to, or being absorbed in a game she was playing with her friends. ADHD just didn't seem to be the right diagnosis, but in the meantime, Sarah was wandering around the classroom and was starting to disrupt the class.

So Sarah's mother knew something was 'off,' but didn't know what.

The Talk to God approach set out in this book is not about diagnosing specific issues, it's about finding out what's really going on under the surface, and trying to decode the spiritual messages God is continually sending us via our health.

The first thing I did was to ask if Sarah had any allergies. The presence of allergies is always a big red sign that the energy in Spleen Meridian is weak, and if the Spleen Meridian is weak, it's very hard for anyone (in this instance, Sarah) to metabolize the new knowledge and information they are receiving from their external environment.

We hit the jackpot: Sarah had a number of food allergies, as well as severe hay fever. Next, I asked if Sarah had an easy or difficult birth (because traumatic circumstances or shock can wipe out Spleen energy in an instant, making it an uphill battle for the body to cope with its food and environment until the energy in the Spleen Meridian has been restored).

Again, jackpot! Sarah's mother had been in labor for 28 hours, the birth had been extremely difficult, and baby Sarah had swallowed a lot of meconium and had been whisked away by the attending doctors as soon as she was born to get it all flushed out.

Next, I asked if Sarah spent a lot of time in front of the big screen, either on the computer or watching TV.

Again, jackpot! Electromagnetic energy can potentially be another huge disrupter of the energy in the Spleen Meridian, as can any other environmental pollutant.

The last question was a lot more sensitive: Was the environment in Sarah's house usually relaxed and encouraging, or more on the stressed and frustrated side of things?

To her credit, Sarah's mother admitted that she was working full time, and with three small children to care for (Sarah was the oldest), she was usually pretty wound-up and tense when she was home. One of the reasons Sarah watched films every day after school was so her mother could have some space to unwind and make supper. (Often, something she could just pull out of the freezer and throw in the oven. Sarah's mother rarely had time to cook much from scratch.)

We started to piece all the bits of the puzzle together, and this is what we got:

The Spleen Meridian is responsible for being able to learn and assimilate new ideas. I believe that together with Triple Warmer, it's the main meridian affecting most learning difficulties.

Spleen energy is associated with compassion and it's weakened by environmental pollutants, shock or trauma, electromagnetic energy, junk food and a negative or stressful emotional environment.

Sarah appeared to be struggling on almost all of those fronts. I suggested some standard energy exercises to start strengthening the Spleen Meridian, which would definitely help, but it looked like there also had to be some changes in Sarah's environment. Sarah's mother left our session with some very big decisions to think about.

As the pressure from the school mounted, she took the plunge and started trying to clean up the family's eating habits. Next, Sarah's mother realized that it was impossible to give Sarah the time and attention she really needed unless she cut back her work.

It was a hard decision, but after a lot of consideration, Sarah's mother went part-time. Now, she had time to take Sarah for weekly sessions with a remedial reading teacher, and within six months, Sarah started to reap the benefits of her mother's self-sacrifice. Now that she was eating more home-cooked food, spending less time in front of the computer, and having a more relaxed home environment and emotionally-available mother, Sarah's marks had improved so much, she was now near the top of the class, and reading voraciously.

Within a year, the 'ADHD' diagnosis had disappeared, and the school stopped pressuring Sarah's mother to put her daughter on Ritalin.

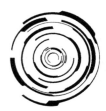

www.spiritualselfhelp.org - The main website for the Jewish Emotional Health Institute (JEMI), where you'll find a wealth of free resources, including:

The 'Talk to God and Fix Your Health' online course - which can help you to translate what you've learned about in this book into solid improvements in your healthcare.

E-books – including: "The Causes and Cures of Depression"; "Guide to Basic Mind-Mapping Techniques"; "The Spiritual Dimension of Healthcare"; "The How, What and Why of Talking to God", and many more.

JEMI's Knowledge Base and popular Blog - regularly updated with the latest on God-based holistic health techniques for healing mind, body and soul.

www.talktogod.today - Lots of practical tips, ideas, discussions and true stories about talking to God.

Energy Medicine Resources on the Web

www.innersource.net - The main website of Donna Eden, author of the bestselling "Energy Medicine" and "Energy Medicine for Women."

www.tatlife.com - The official website for the Tapas Acupressure Technique (TAT)

www.emofree.com - Website of Gary Craig, the founder of the 'Emotional Freedom' Tapping Technique

Recommended Reading

BOOKS FOR THE BODY

Energy Medicine: Balancing Your Body's Energies for Optimal Health, Joy and Vitality - By Donna Eden and David Feinstein, PhD

The Body Electric: Electromagnetism and the Foundation of life - Robert Becker, MD and Gary Seldon.

Vibrational Medicine: The No.1 Handbook of Subtle-Energy Therapies - Richard Gerber, MD

Energy Medicine: The Scientific Basis - James L. Oschman

The Natural Recovery Plan: Chronic Fatigue, ME and Fibromyalgia - Alison Adams

Spontaneous Healing: How to discover and enhance your body's natural ability to maintain and heal itself - Andrew Weil, MD

Pharmageddon: (An expose of the modern pharmaceutical industry) - David Healy

Touch for Health: A Practical Guide to Natural Health with Acupressure Touch - John Thie, DC and Matthew Thie, M.Ed

BOOKS FOR THE MIND

The Happy Workshop: An eight week journey to real, lasting happiness - Rivka Levy

Running on Empty: Overcome your childhood emotional neglect - Jonice Webb

Aromatherapy for Healing the Spirit: Restoring emotional and mental balance with essential oils - Gabriel Mojay

The Promise of Energy Psychology: Gary Craig, David Feinstein and Donna Eden and Gary Craig

The Ultimate You: Using *emuna* to break through personal barriers - Dr Zev Ballen

BOOKS FOR THE SOUL

The Garden of Emuna: A practical guide to life - Shalom Arush

Connection: Emotional and spiritual growth through experiencing God's presence - Efim Svirsky

Healing Words: The power of prayer, and the practice of medicine - Larry Dossey, MD

Index

Symbols

About the Author

My name's Rivka Levy, and I'm a widely-published journalist and writer of 20 years' standing. I've authored five books broadly about spiritual self-help and holistic health, including: 'The Happy Workshop' and 'Causes and Cures of Depression'. I also founded the Jewish Emotional Health Institute (JEMI), which is devoted to giving people practical, easy tools for how to use God-based holistic health techniques to transform their mind, body and soul.

Before changing track to God-based holistic health, I owned my own PR firm in London, U.K. and before that, I was a top ghostwriter for some of the biggest names in the British government. The deadlines and pressure nearly killed me, and I burned out at the age of 35, moved to Israel, and started looking for some real, spiritual answers to many of the health and personal issues I was facing in my own life.

For a while, I couldn't even so much as look at a keyboard, and I thought I was going to becoming a holistic health practitioner instead. I did course after course, and got officially certified as an aromatherapist, *emuna* spiritual coach and energy medicine practitioner specializing in the link between Chinese Energy Medicine and emotions.

While I was learning all this stuff, I started to piece together a much bigger, holistic health paradigm that explained how happiness, holiness and health really fit together. Enough time had passed for me to return to my keyboard, and I realized that I could help far more people by writing books about what was really causing their health issues, and how to really resolve them, than I could by doing one-on-one sessions.

Now, I'm on a mission to transform the way people relate to their own health and happiness by helping them make the connections between their own physical health, their feelings, and their spiritual dimension in a non-weird, scientifically-proven way.

I write for a number of publications, maintain three blogs and also lecture extensively about the God-based holistic approach to happiness and health.

If you have any questions, comments or feedback about this book, I'd love to hear from you. Please drop me a line at: rivkawritesback@gmail.com

THANKS FOR READING THIS BOOK!

If you enjoyed it, please take a moment to give it
an online review at any of the following sites:

www.amazon.com

www.goodreads.com

www.booktalk.org

www.shelfari.com

www.bookpage.com

www.librarything.com

CPSIA information can be obtained
at www.ICGtesting.com
Printed in the USA
LVOW03s1459100616

492101LV00007B/108/P